HÉCTOR ROSSO

Spiritual Awakening of a Nurse

From the Death of a Child to Loving Kindness

LOTUS
LIBRARY

SPIRITUAL AWAKENING OF A NURSE;
From the Death of a Child to Loving Kindness

First published in Great Britain in 2019 by Lotus Library
Copyright ©Héctor Rosso, 2019

The moral right of the author has been asserted.

A CIP catalogue record for this book is available from the British Library.

ISBN 978-1-7331232-4-2

Managing Editor for Lotus Library: Julie Watson
Developmental Editor: Jennifer Watson Ervedosa
Translation from Spanish to English: Flor Taboada www.flortaboada.com
Cover Design, typesetting and internal illustrations © Clare Connie Shepherd
www.clareconnieshepherd.com
Internal artwork ©Julie Watson www.saatchiart.com/juliewatson

Lotus Library is an imprint of Watson Caring Science Institute, a 501C(3) international non-profit foundation.

Watson Caring Science Institute, 4450 Arapahoe Avenue Suite 100, Boulder, CO 80303 USA
www.watsoncaringscience.org

LOTUS
LIBRARY

Watson Caring
Science Institute

HÉCTOR ROSSO

Spiritual Awakening of a Nurse

From the Death
of a Child to
Loving Kindness

LOTUS
LIBRARY

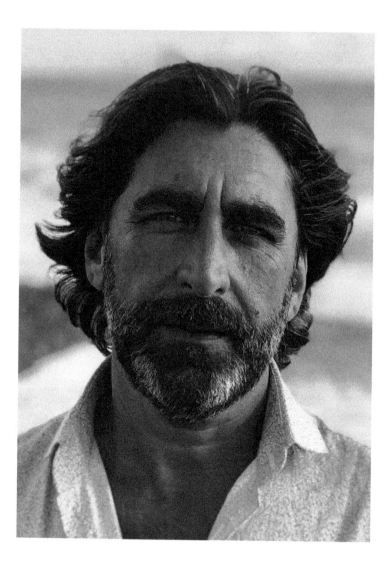

About the author

Héctor Rosso RN, BSN, CDE, MA,
CARITAS COACH®,
Faculty Associate, Watson Caring Science Institute

A native of Montevideo, Héctor Rosso worked as a nurse in Uruguay for more than 28 years.

He was Professor and Director at the Department for Education & Community Health, Faculty of Nursing & Health Technologies, at Catholic University, Uruguay, and more recently, he was Assistant Director of a large psychiatric hospital, in addition to serving as Director of Nursing at the only Public pediatric hospital in Uruguay. This experience deepened his desire to develop well-being and care for nurses, which formulated his research for his double Master's thesis, completed in 2018. Currently, Héctor is an Adjunct Faculty Associate for WCSI, and a Caring Science Scholar, committed to a leading role on "WCSI Sur," supporting Spanish speaking health professionals interested in Caring Science. Héctor also works as a holistic nurse educator, speaker, and consultant; and is honored to support nurses and other care givers with their own personal and professional development.

He is also a certified Reiki Practitioner.

Hector currently divides his time between Hollywood, Florida and Brighton, England, where he enjoys taking long walks on the beach while listening to love songs from the 80s in the company of his beloved "mate"(traditional tea).

This is his first book.

Foreword

By Jean Watson

As we trust life and death as a sacred circle, a never-ending circle for humanity, and our human experiences on the Mother Earth plane, we long for meaningful purpose and depth to face all the pain and despair in our inner and outer world. As we do so, through our own journey, we discover that we are all faced with human tasks of healing our relationship with self and other; finding new meaning in human suffering, searching for deeper meaning of life and, ultimately, facing our own death and those closest to us. Through this never ending universal sacred circle of life/death/rebirth – through the story of another who has opened his heart with this life-death passage, we have a personal map toward finding new meaning and even purpose beyond.

Héctor Rosso shares his personal/professional life journey through such an artistic and authentic story that it invites others to enter deep healing experiences, literally and vicariously.

Any parent who has lost a child will be made more whole and wiser, during and after experiencing this personal expose of self-healing. It provides an inner and outer search for self/ soul through an experiential passage of loss, grief, death, despair, chaos, confusion, and suffering – finally surrendering to deep healing and transformation. A quest for solutions led to travels to another country where dwelling in meditative, contemplative quieting of the suffering mind, resulted in higher deeper consciousness – in what one may consider a soul-retrieval.

Any person who has experienced death of a loved one; any health professional who works with loss, grief, death of a child or family member, will be more able to grasp the inner continuous painful, soulless journey of a parent's loss, despair, and helplessness, with ultimate finality of living through death itself. On the other side of this passage is the process which led to a new wave of freedom from pain; a new sense and surrender to the beauty and mysteries of life with a future, not imagined.

Jean Watson, PhD, RN, AHN-BC, FAAN, LL (AAN)
Founder/Director Watson Caring Science InstituteBoulder, Colorado USA
Distinguished Professor Dean Emerita University of Colorado Denver,
College of Nursing
Recipient of 15 Honorary Doctorates (12 International) American
Academy of Nursing Living Legend - 2013

Foreword

By Erika Caballero Muñoz

In times of armed conflicts, environmental changes, chronic health issues, life and death, this book is a balm for the soul, a way to find ourselves and our divine love essence again in a sacred universe.

This book is the account of a nurse and the profound personal discovery of himself and his essence through commitment, love and gratitude to his soul teacher, his daughter Julieta.

It is a guide to support parents who, plunged into the pain of losing a child, must be reborn, but it also points out a way for health professionals and the need to ground their work in a philosophy and a caring science.

The book you are holding in your hands will show you the way in which a man became more human through the infinitive love of his children and family and through spiritual development in harmonious connection with the universe. This book substantiates the discovery of a former healing path through our ancestors, a path that they followed and that will always forge our own spiritual path towards a holistic view.

Each of the paragraphs describing the experiences of the author and my dear friend will help you as a professional discover the ways to heal and accompany children in their suffering, and throughout their palliative care. The learning is just to be, but also to give ourselves permission to be taken care of and be open to oneself and to the caring situation, as proposed by Jean Watson.

This book will take you on a path that will allow you to connect with yourself, bringing together your head, your heart and your hands and translating through them loving care practices. You will be taken into a journey of discovering that caring is a sacred act, an act of love where each caring moment is unique and must be lived as such by being present for the other. It will take you on a path of forgiveness, gratitude and true healing.

Through this beautiful book, you will be able to rediscover the meaning of honoring death and acknowledging that we die in each moment, in the sense that each breath allows us to experience, as Watson points out, the miracle of life, because death is a sacred wheel of life.

Héctor's trip to Paraguay shows us brilliantly the importance of a regular contemplative and meditative practice to provide equanimity, love and goodness to oneself and to others, and to allow a connection with life's transpersonal dimension. With this trip, he invites us to acknowledge the importance of forgiveness and gratitude as a means to clean our soul. He teaches us to experience loss as a transformative act. The book walks us through the 10 Caritas Processes® which are the guiding light of the act of caring.

I'm grateful to my dear friend for his courage to capture in this book his life experiences because he, as myself, have both been blessed with a path that freed us into miracles by opening us up to Caritas and the loving practice of centering and taking care of ourselves and others with healing intent. He leaves us a Life lesson that enables us to understand the Caring Science, that allows us to say "I am when we are" connected in an energetic field of love and deep healing.

Erika Caballero Muñoz

Nurse - Midwife

Magister Instructional Design

High Risk Newborn Nursing Specialist

Expert in Informatics in Nursing and Distance Education

UVISA Academic Director

Board Member of the International Council of Nurses (Region 6)

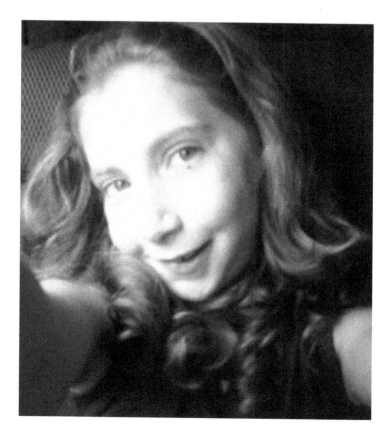

Julieta Rosso
06-07-2000 / 19-10-2013

Dedication

To the memory of my beautiful and sweet daughter Julieta Rosso, relentless fighter, teacher of life, eternal joy, boundless happiness, feast of smiles, extraordinary daughter, better sister and friend, great lover of animals and nature …

Acknowledgements

To my children, Lucia and Enzo Rosso, for their support, unconditional love, and source of inspiration in this life.

To my sweet wife Julie Watson, companion in my new life and a great woman.

To Jean Watson for her vision of a better world and for empowering the nursing profession to act as a sacred assignment, and for her legacy of Caring Science – a gift to the world.

To Lynne Wagner, my teacher and mentor during my Caritas Coach Education Program® (CCEP), a great colleague and friend.

To Jan Anderson for her wise teachings.

To Erika Caballero, a great friend, spiritual guide and professional. Thank you for your support and the healing given to Julieta during the most difficult of times.

To life and the eternal energy of the Universe …

"Just as in our personal lives during crisis or illness, tragedy, loss, or imminent death, we ponder spiritual questions that go beyond the physical material world; it is here in our evolving professional-scientific life that we may need to ponder new meanings.

In our conventional,
dispirited, physical-
technical life form,
deathbed of sorts,
Caring Science offers
new freedom, new space
to reconsider a deeper
meaning of caring-
healing of work
and phenomena."
(Watson, 2005, p. 139)

Author's Foreword

On love, death and healing – writing for self and others

This book was born out of my own personal experience of losing a child which is one of the most difficult situations a human being can go through.

This is a journey of love, loss, suffering, and healing framed within Jean Watson's Theory of Caring Science.

This is a book to help guide parents and health professionals who have been or are going through, loss and healing. It is based on my own personal life experience, and my experience as a professional nurse through the lens of Caring Science.

I discovered my spiritual path during a time of profound suffering after caring for and losing my daughter, Julieta, who was diagnosed with cancer when she was 6 years old. She died when she was 13 after having endured years of challenging treatments, and a little over a year of palliative care.

During this profound spiritual search, I encountered several different holistic disciplines and began to study Watson's Theory of Caring Science and the 10 Caritas Processes®. My healing started while I was training as a Watson Caring

Science Caritas Coach®. At the time, I imagined that the writing of this book would help me process my own healing and could help other parents in similar situations.

This book describes my life and my relationship with myself, my daughter, and my family as well as the discovery of my true essence and transformation into a more spiritually alive being.

This is the beginning of a path to deepen my understanding and expansion of my own self-healing and the healing of others as a Caritas Coach.

The aim of this book, guided by Caring Science, is that it will be a healing touchstone for family members who have endured the loss of a child and for health professionals who play a part in care and treatment of these families.

In particular, the book is for parents going through a similar situation: for siblings, grandparents, uncles and aunts, (members of the extended family) and their communities. It is for nurses and other health professionals, both conventional and/or complementary. I believe Caring Science has the power to help anyone who cares about living, dying, and grieving.

This book has been developed, planned, and written from the heart through the eyes and reflection of a father and nurse who suffered. My aim is that it will serve as a reference, a tool and guide for healing. It is an honest and personal experience that I hope will provide advice and guidance to those who experience illness, to those caring for the terminally ill in palliative care, and for those with an interest in death and dying, grief, and loss. It is an example of resilience and life after death. It is about relationships and family challenges.

It is also a guide for professionals, a way to see an example of the human side of disease and loss through the lens of Caring Science and Caritas.

My purpose is to be creative and artistic in a personal and thoughtful way, guiding the reader through transpersonal connections, encouraging compassion and love for oneself and others in the healing process.

It is a self-reflective deeply personal book, with me as a writer and person at its center.

I left my country, Uruguay, with the sole purpose of focusing on studying Caring Science and the English language in order to understand the theory better (since the majority of the work is written in English).

Using Caring Science as my guiding principle and weaving the 10 Caritas Processes throughout my experience, I have developed the framework and content of my book.

Through self-reflection, first about the years of my life I spent caring for my daughter with cancer, and later years working through my sorrow, I have organised my thoughts by drawing a timeline with key chronological moments which have formed the foundation of the chapters of this book. In these chapters you will find different notes: "Caritas reflections" or "Caring Science quotes" which are for parents/ family members, and for nurses/health professionals who may want to reflect on Human Caring values.

This book is written in Spanish and translated into English. It is divided into four chapters which describe my everyday life events and my transformative experiences.

Table of Contents

CHAPTER III   The two 'intermediate years' or
years of my denial, my indifference
and effort to keep going in a
robotic way. I was focusing only
on my work, studying, and my
financial responsibilities without
honoring my great loss or the pain
and need for self-care and healing.
This chapter includes my solo
trip to Paraguay, an event
where I experienced a profound
confrontation with myself that
changed my life. With great agony
I faced the reality of a broken
heart – an immense raw pain
– and I surrendered fully to my
sorrow. In Paraguay I developed
a relationship with grief which
allowed me to focus on myself and
my own needs for the first time.

CHAPTER IV A new perspective and awareness
of the self, deep loss, and the
need for healing. I began my
soul-searching journey and my
heart changed. The process
of honoring my authentic self
and acknowledging our deep
connection with the universe
gave rise to the discovery of
my true self. Only through this
incorporation of a new and
deeper healing was I able to
invite Caring Science to me, to
lead me to Caritas so that I was
able to become a Caritas Coach.
A change of life, a time for
forgiveness, love, gratitude
and vulnerability.

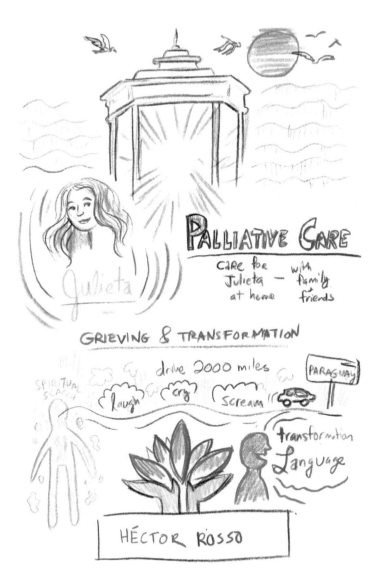

PALLIATIVE CARE

care for Julieta at home — with family friends

Julieta

GRIEVING & TRANSFORMATION

SPIRITUAL SEARCH

drive 2000 miles

laugh   cry   scream

PARAGUAY

transformation Language

HÉCTOR ROSSO

Chapter I

A new path

Today is the beginning of a new path, the path of writing about my life, about my anecdotes, about fond moments as well as about painful and very sorrowful moments. But all of them (happy and painful) have ultimately brought me to life teachings that have made me who I am today.

I can say with certainty that today I consider myself a man who is much more aware of his humanness. I am filled with love and have a goal: to continue walking my path of searching, in order to deepen my spiritual life and to help those around me. I want to continue to experience profound and harmonious contact with the universe and explore the many facets of connecting with the divine/energy of the universe. Call it Reiki, Akashic records, yoga, meditation, walking the labyrinth, shamanic energy, the Uruguayan Path of the Children of Earth, sacred ancestral medicine, Caritas, Tibetan bowls, de-coding, talking with the Angels, God, etc. To me these all have the same goal: connecting with oneself/ the divine/the universe/love.

This new way of life that I have undertaken with total freedom and consciousness is completely opposite to the life I had before. In the past, spirituality wasn't my thing at all. I only believed what I could see, in what could be scientifically proven. But today I'm convinced that this is my new way to live, in total communion with my essence, with my inner self and the universe.

There is a branch of my family that has always had a big connection with spirituality, especially my paternal great grandfather and my great aunt. I had the honor to live with this aunt for many years when I was a child. Lovingly, we used to call her "Auntie Peti." She was the healer in the neighborhood. Neighbors and acquaintances would come to her looking for help. At the time, I was making my first forays into nursing and I viewed these situations with a degree of skepticism. Now looking back, I appreciate the important role she played in our community, and the great deal of support she selflessly offered to many people. Without a doubt, she was my first holistic teacher. Today, I realise how important a figure she is in my life because, amongst other things, she forged the opening of my spiritual path.

Onset of, and navigation through, Julieta's illness

My spiritual awakening began with the painful death of my little daughter, the youngest of my three children. The beautiful Julieta was my great teacher. She taught me about life, strength, love, surrender, union, goodness, joy, pain, sorrow, about hard times but even more so about good times and great times.

Julieta was an exceptional human being with a unique energy. She managed to overcome many kinds of chemotherapies, surgeries, and radiotherapy sessions (not only once but several times), with all that this entails.

At the beginning of Julieta's illness, our family situation was strained because it had been a year since I had separated with Cecilia, the mother of my children. At first this made the situation more complicated, but later things began to move more harmoniously for the sake of Julieta's care and well-being.

The onset of the illness occurred at the end of 2006, and initially we thought she was incubating a parotitis (most commonly known as mumps). Unfortunately, it didn't turn out to be something as benign as that. On the 23rd of December of that year, (the day before Christmas Eve), the cancer diagnoses arrived (Rhabdomyosarcoma of parotid gland). It is impossible to forget that Christmas full of uncertainty and pain.

Julieta was only 6 years old and had just finished her first year at school. From now on, her life would be accompanied by her illness – the cancer – until her death.

At her school play for the New Year's party in December of 2006, Julieta was thrilled to be cast as the lead role in Mary Poppins. It was something that had a great impact on her. It brought so much joy and happiness to her that we used to watch the film during times when the treatment was most painful. Watching the film was for her a way to escape and be transported to a place of joy and happiness. It was very beautiful and moving to see her watching her favorite film.

As I write this paragraph, I have been transported to the feelings of love and wholeness of that time and, each time I read it, it happens again. It is a bittersweet feeling, one that brings tightness to my chest …

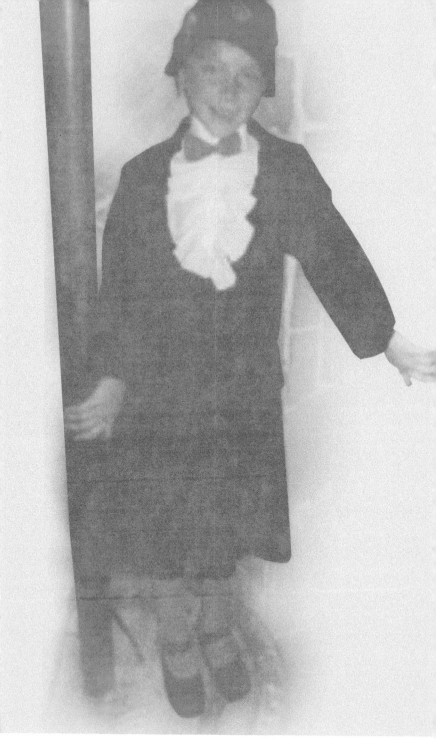

The first round of chemotherapy
and the surgery

After the 2006 Christmas holiday, the chemotherapy began. For approximately six weeks, they bombarded her with everything.

The chemotherapy was very strong, and the side effects didn't take long to appear such as vomiting, nausea, discomfort, and weakness. We endured long sessions at the hospital outpatient department (sometimes eight to ten hours). But Julieta was very strong and positive. Once back at home she would recover quickly in the company of her friends, pets, and family.

In February 2007 after long chemotherapy sessions, surgery was performed on Julieta in the Centro Hospitalario Pereira Rossell in Montevideo, Uruguay. This hospital had been my place of work for over 15 years. The surgery was planned with the ENT Professor, (an excellent person and professional who always supported us both as a doctor and as a human being). Alongside this doctor, there was a maxillofacial odontologist surgeon and a multidisciplinary team of professionals. The surgery lasted well over eight hours, not including the pre-operative and the post-operative care.

Being a nurse myself, I always had the opportunity to be next to Julieta, even in the operating theater. With my company I was able to help her gain confidence and feel safe until she fell asleep. I would stay with her until she was fully anaesthetised. It was very important for her that I was there by her side so that she didn't get nervous. I would also be in the operating theater or recovery room before she woke up waiting for her.

I'm grateful to all of my co-workers on the Pediatric Hospital Surgery Team for their exceptional and very caring work.

My feelings during this period are indescribable. I was overwhelmed, devastated. I couldn't believe this was happening – even less so being a health professional myself and thus understanding a little more than most of what was yet to come. But I couldn't express my feelings. I needed to be the solid support of my family – for my other two children, Lucia and Enzo, and for the mother of my children. Throughout Juli's illness I always felt I had to remain strong and show endurance. There wasn't any time for me.

Who cares for the Carer?

" One of the first
requirements for stepping
into a model of caring-
healing and Caritas
Consciousness is to
be fully present in the
moment, more open
and available to self
and situation."
(Watson, 2008, p. 54)

Now with hindsight, I realise how committed and dedicated I was to others always making sure that everyone else was fine. But what happened to me? I don't regret my role at all, on the contrary, I'd do it again if necessary. But I'd do it with a different wisdom, with the awareness that self-care and love is the way, the tool, the most powerful ally.

During this time, I was lucky to have by my side an exceptional woman, Laura, who gave me protection, help and support. She was (then) my partner and her support continued for many years after. She is a beautiful person and I'm eternally grateful to her for having been my companion during the most difficult time in my life. It was a collective resilience. Juli was like a daughter to Laura, and Juli's parting was very painful for her too.

The first round of radiotherapy

After Julieta's surgery, the radiotherapy treatment began. We went for treatment Monday to Friday for several weeks. It was complicated because each time we visited the healthcare team had to make a special mask for her before she could even begin to undergo the radiotherapy session. It must be taken into account that we are talking about a 6-year-old child having just endured a very complex chemotherapy experience and a long recovery from surgery. Despite everything, Julieta faced it all with great courage.

I remember the radiotherapy took place in the winter, and one of the things Juli most liked to do after the radiotherapy sessions was to eat "tortas fritas" from a street vendor. "Tortas fritas" is a typical Uruguayan food, eaten in winter or on rainy days. It is a kind of bread made of flour, water and salt, and fried in fat. Juli was so happy with so little …

Her face wasn't the same anymore. The surgery had left its mark and the radiotherapy didn't help with the recovery process – quite the opposite – as it had damaged her skin. I remember we had to apply a special cream often to her skin. It didn't take long for the onset of the alopecia. It was a challenge on its own to watch her beautiful long blond curly hair fall out, to see such a lovely girl with a completely different face and without her hair.

"We emanate our presence and radiate from our heart center in a given caring moment. But our presence can be head-centered or heart-centered, or we can unite head and heart and actions to connect with the infinity of Love …" (Watson, 2005, p. 115)

Incredibly, she overcame all of these treatments and little by little began to return to her routine like attending school and taking part in her hobbies. That year was very hard. All our hopes were set on Juli's illness ending there and then. The days went by as did the medical checks, with their customary blood tests, CT scans, etcetera, etcetera; all of which were taking a great deal of time away from her short childhood.

The recurrence of the cancer

Two years had passed since the onset of Juli's illness. We were feeling relieved that everything had ended and was behind us. Unfortunately, that didn't turn out to be the case.

Our excitement and happiness were abruptly cut short.

One of the CT scans showed a new cancer, a recurrence. Previously, the cancer had been located in the right upper maxilla, where the parotid had been removed. Now the recurrence was following along the inferior maxilla towards her mouth. We were back to square one with one difference: the chances of a cure were now much reduced. The consultants told us surgery would be very complex, and they didn't know how best to approach it because in Uruguay there wasn't much expertise in this particular kind of surgery.

From that point onwards a restless search began. Where could the surgery be performed, and what would the cost be to have it done abroad? We approached several universities and hospitals in the USA, Argentina, and Brazil, but time was pressing on and we had to find a solution and a suitable treatment soon!

We decided that a consultation at the Hospital Sirio-Libanés in São Paulo, Brazil, was the best option. This hospital is a benchmark in South America, with a reputation in the field of cancer surgery and treatment.

So off we went, Julieta, her mother and I, for a series of initial consultations with the doctors, pediatric oncologist, maxillofacial and plastic surgeons.

In the beginning, I remember how everything was new to Juli – it was the first time she had flown on a plane. We had a really special time enjoying little moments with great happiness and forgetting (for a while) about the illness. The consultations reassured us that we were going to find a solution. The plastic surgeon told us that this was going to be a big challenge for him because Juli's face had been so badly affected by the previous surgery, the chemo, the radio, and now by the new tumor. One of the three doctors spoke Spanish, so we were able to understand each other. We returned to Uruguay with high hopes and ready to face whatever was coming our way during this new stage of the illness.

Some days after our return from São Paulo we were informed of the cost of Juli's new surgery. This was a whole new chapter in our new treatment process. Each doctor had very high fees of thousands of US dollars, and in addition there was the need for everything else such as travel, food and accommodation in Brazil. And this was just the cost of our first surgery!

We needed to secure the funding as soon as possible and so began our monumental quest to find it.

We received amazing support from many people: social organisations, unions, companies and institutions, neighbors, co-workers, friends, family, and even people we didn't know all generously supported our fundraising campaign to accomplish Julieta's surgery abroad. For Julieta this was a marathon.

We will always be eternally grateful especially to our community for their invaluable support and solidarity.

Money was collected and various artistic events organised in order to raise funds. We received many donations, we organised TV, radio, and social media campaigns. Our family and close friends worked tirelessly to raise the money we needed to start without delay.

The second surgery (Brazil)

The truth is that we went back to São Paulo to have the surgery with only a third of the money required, just enough to get us started. The treatment couldn't wait so we jumped! Finances were an additional stress that at times became unbearable. But we needed to face it and carry on.

We bought plane tickets and arranged accommodation in a hotel opposite the hospital. There was going to be just the two of us (with Julieta) and we needed a place nearby to eat, wash, and once she was discharged, a place to be with Julieta during the recovery process that was located near to the Outpatient Department.

For my other children, Lucia and Enzo, this was a very tough and challenging time, as they spent long periods away from their parents and their sister. Naturally they were well cared for and protected by their maternal family, who gave them support and loving care. However, being in their early teens, they also had to face the pain and anguish of their sister's illness at a distance from their parents due to the treatment of their sister abroad. It was also tough because Julieta was taking all of our attention.

In the creation of this book, different memories of that time come to mind, and I'd like to share a very special one that really touched me and filled me with great love.

As I began to remember details of times living with Julieta, some experiences are still very present and real, so much so that the other day while I was meditating on the beach in Brighton (England), I had a memory so vivid that it felt as though I was watching a movie of Julieta's delivery and birth. In a flash of a second, I saw the whole event. I remembered with much love and joy every detail from the initial prenatal check-ups and the moment Cecilia went into labor, to the hospital and the arrival of our beautiful baby without any complications. I then remembered the day we introduced Julieta to Lucia and Enzo, who were 3 and 2 years old at the time. It fills me with an instant great joy. Those were very beautiful years. I appreciate the memories of those three lovely children growing up together.

At the time, Cecilia and I were working as Scouts volunteers. We were educators in the Padre Jacinto Tuccillo Scout Group No 6. I remember this period of our lives very clearly. I'm proud of the way we shared with our children our connection to, and love for nature. Together we camped in many pretty places around our country with endless activities such as bonfires, walks, starry nights, and going for swims in the sea and rivers. All the while surrounded by beautiful people; adults and educators, parent helpers, children, teenagers and the beneficiary youngsters whom we were training. These moments are unforgettable and leave a mark that lasts forever. They are memories full of beauty, love, peace, goodness, brotherhood and sisterhood and joy achieved simply – with a tent and a backpack the adventure was guaranteed! They were great family moments.

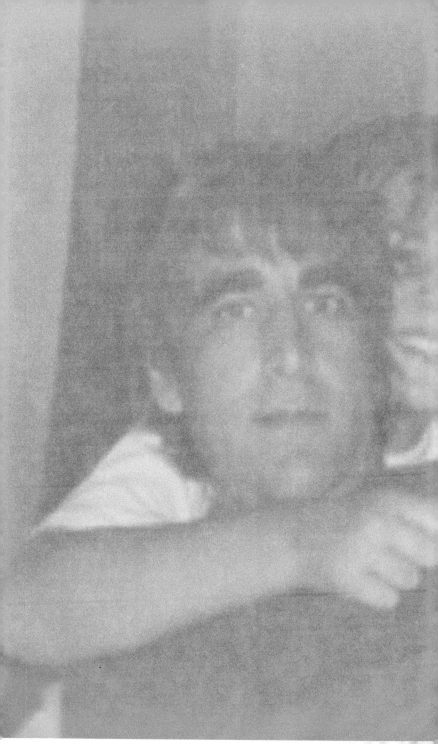

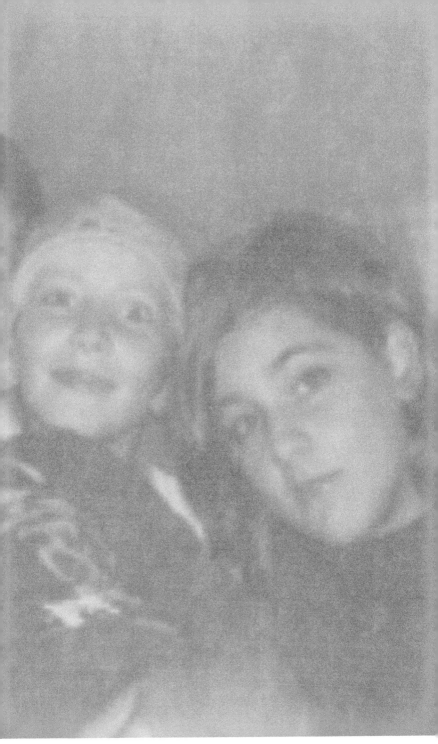

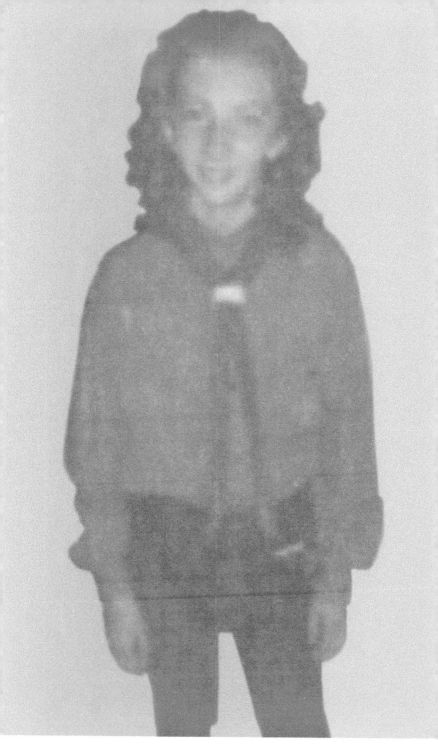

On the day of the Julieta's surgery in São Paulo we were anxious. We knew it was going to be difficult, especially the recovery. Being in a foreign country without speaking the language was challenging for us but especially hard for Julieta, however the lovely Brazilians treated us very well and we had a lot of support from the health professionals and others around us. For Julieta – to be far away from the things she most loved like her siblings, her home and the rest of her family, friends, neighborhood, toys, pets, her entire world – was terribly difficult.

The first day in São Paulo began in an entertaining and happy way. The room at the Hospital Sirio Libanés was beautiful, uplifting and welcoming. It was a private room unlike the rooms in Uruguay (where she had always shared her room with other children). The preoperative care had begun the day before with the routine procedures: hygiene, blood tests, putting in place the PVC (vein catheters), and the appropriate diet plan agreed in order to start the fasting. I remember she was fascinated, as though nothing was going to happen the next day.

Without a doubt she, like us, was anxious and had set her hopes on the success of the surgery to remove the tumor and on the reconstruction. They were going to use part of her peronei (leg) and surrounding muscle for the reconstruction of her inferior maxilla after the removal of the tumor. Who knows what her face and leg were going to look like?

The day of the surgery began with me (as always) by her side. She said goodbye to her mum at the entrance of the operating theatre while I went to get changed into scrubs in order to go in with her. Facing a surgery without being able to understand the language of the nurses and doctors was an additional stress, particularly for a little girl, but thanks to my profession I could be next to her because I understood the rules and protocols of an operating theater. This was really important for us because I was able to support her so that she felt safe and secure.

I want to thank all the staff who never had any objections and understood that it was necessary for me to be with her. This was a very humane Caritas act on the part of the assisting medical team.

Julieta and I had a very close and deep relationship, particularly when she was feeling vulnerable and facing the adversity of her health challenges. As soon as she began to feel better however, she had that same close and deep relationship with her mother. This is why it was so important for her to be able to count on the both of us.

The surgery was a great success, and everything went according to plan. Now was the beginning of a long period of recovery. We stayed at the hospital for several days. The recovery was going to be slow and long, and we had to face a number of challenges. There were mobility issues due to the big wound on her leg. Julieta wasn't able to walk and so had to move around in a wheelchair. Eating was also a challenge. This could only be done through nasogastric intubation. How she was going to talk was also a big challenge. She was going to be tracheostomised for a long period of time (a tracheostomy is a surgical procedure where an opening is created through the neck and a catheter inserted in order to allow the passage of air to the lungs). It became necessary to teach Julieta what to do herself in order to be able to talk and communicate. All this without our forgetting about the importance of care – the dressing of her surgical wounds, etc.

After she was discharged, we continued the recovery process in the hotel which wasn't easy since it didn't have the right infrastructure for patient recovery. However, we adjusted and managed this well, putting into it lots of our love and enthusiasm, so Julieta could recover her health and feel ready to travel back to Uruguay as soon as possible.

For her, it was very important to enjoy a variety of leisure and game-oriented activities in order to manage her own recovery. She liked painting, writing stories, playing with her toys, table tennis, card games and watching DVDs of her favorite films. In the middle of her recovery process, we felt it was appropriate to go to São Paulo's zoo because Juli really enjoyed and missed contact with nature. It was an incredible experience that helped to lift her spirits a great deal. We spent several hours having fun and enjoying ourselves without thinking about the many procedures of the treatment.

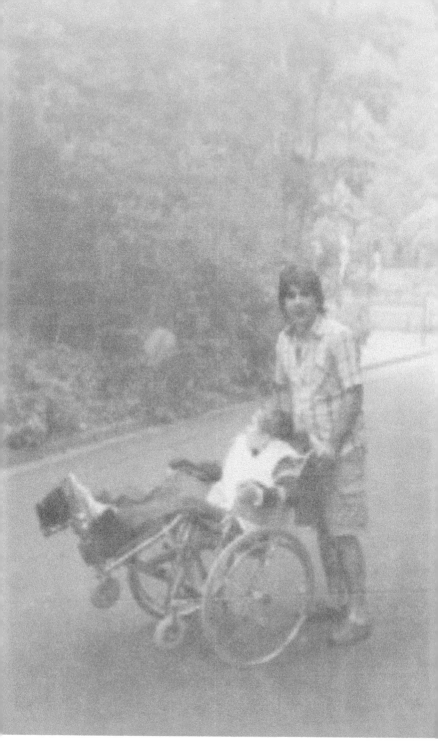

Return to Montevideo

We returned to Uruguay to start the chemotherapy again which would last for several months.

Julieta had to face (again) a long and hard treatment with (again) many complications. It was during this time we decided to support her care with complementary therapies. We did lots of alternative treatments to complement Julieta's health, including Homeopathy.

One treatment in particular required financial effort and time spent traveling and consulting with doctors in Cuba on a new natural product called Escozul (a Cuban traditional medicine) that is currently being researched to treat cancer. As a parent, one turns to all possible methods and so we decided it was important that Julieta was treated with this product.

I'd like to praise and thank the Cuban Public Health Service for opening their doors to us. The medical team took an interest in Julieta's case and provided both the product and all the procedures free of charge!

Julieta's wish to visit Disney World

My sister Elizabeth was always very supportive of me, despite living far away in another country. She was always there, making her contribution in several ways, but one in particular is engraved in our hearts.

Elizabeth organised a 'Make-a-Wish® campaign.' Make-a-Wish is a global organisation which grants wishes to children living with chronic and/or terminal illnesses.

When Elizabeth started the application process, we were in the midst of treatment in Sao Paulo, and so the Wish came in from their office in Brazil.

Julieta was interviewed on several occasions by representatives of the organisation, and during the interviews she was asked about her wish in order to be assessed for the selection process. Julieta shared her wish: she would like to visit Walt Disney World and share the experience with her Florida auntie, uncle and cousins whom she hadn't seen for many years. And the wish came true! We were able to travel in October 2010, after the chemotherapy treatment in Uruguay had ended. We all traveled there together: her mother, her siblings and me. It was a magical, unforgettable trip, experienced as a family. Julieta enjoyed the moment to the fullest.

Our family is beyond grateful to the amazing Make-a-Wish® organisation which does so much for children suffering all over the world.

At the time, Joaquín, my youngest nephew was four months old. The experience of sharing a week with my sister's family and my nieces and nephews was really special for me and for my three children. Together we enjoyed many beautiful moments. We spent a week at 'Give Kids the World Village®' in Orlando Florida.

There is something I particularly remember from this trip during a day in the 'rapids' at one of Disney's water parks. I recall with much joy the experience of connection with my daughter that morning. Always adventurous, Julieta had the idea of us climbing into and walking through the water rapids. It was one of the main attractions at Disney's water parks and had a long pathway of water which continuously ran at a certain speed. The crazy thing was there were times when we couldn't touch the bottom, and the area of Juli's tracheostomy was still healing! The water was deep and moving at great speed. She really enjoyed it but for me there were times when I was incredibly nervous and worried because I had to keep her afloat and not let go of her under any circumstances (to keep the area of the tracheostomy above water)! To be honest it was hugely stressful for me but, as she was enjoying it so much, seeing her happiness and joy gave me the confidence and security to go for it. I have to confess that I finished the experience with a few skin abrasions in several areas of my body because the sides of the rapids were rugged and rough, and I had to keep Julieta afloat at all times. But seeing Juli's enjoyment and sharing this experience with her made it all worthwhile.

The cancer comes back

After a year of intense living out strenous moments during the treatment, and times of joy during the trip to Disney the cancer came back. There isn't an adjective which could ever possibly describe my feelings. The pain and anguish was overwhelming. But as always, we needed to carry on.

We needed to return to Brazil, but we had run out of financial resources to face the costs for a second time. In the end it was Pedro, the Brazilian doctor, and Julio, the maxillofacial surgeon, who ended up helping us with the paperwork so that Julieta could be admitted into the public hospital system at São Paulo Hospital Público das Clínicas.

We want to graciously thank the Brazilian Public Health System and the fantastic medical team at this hospital.

After the surgery, chemotherapy wasn't an option for us anymore, and so the idea of performing a very specific radiotherapy in the affected area (at the Hospital Sirio-Libanés) was decided upon.

By then we had found the money to cover the costs thanks to the Fundación Peluffo Gigens of Uruguay.

We are very grateful to the Peluffo Gigens Foundation and to the technical team who always supported Julieta.

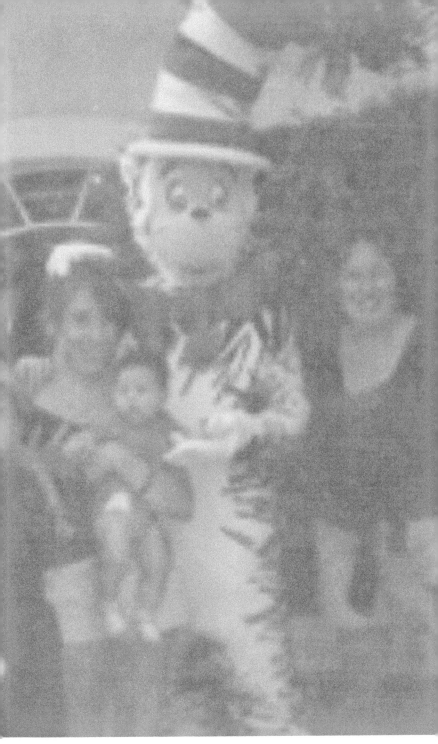

An anecdote from this time was meeting Lula da Silva in the radiotherapy waiting room at the Hospital Sirio-Libanés in São Paulo. Lula shared some time with Julieta. She was fascinated that she had just met the man who up until recently had been the President of Brazil!

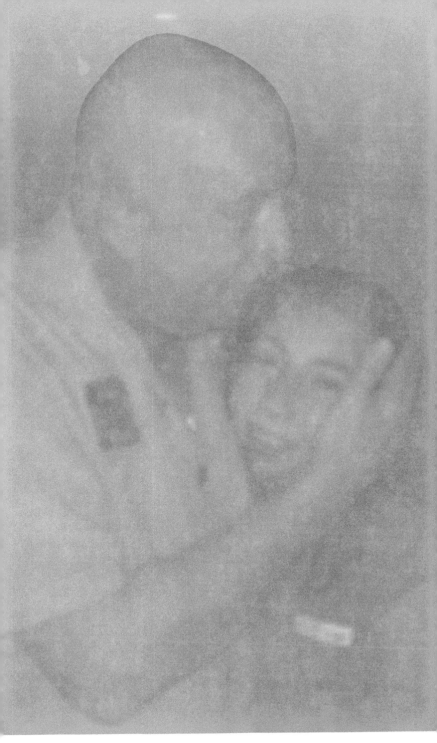

"Effective Caring promotes healing, health, individual/family growth and a sense of wholeness, forgiveness, evolved consciousness, and inner peace that trancends the crisis and fear of disease, diagnosis, illness, traumas, life changes, and so on."
(Watson, 2008, p.17)

"In Caring Science, we can appreciate, honor, and face the reality that life is given to us as a gift; we are invited to sustain and deepen our own and others' humanity as our moral ethical starting point for professional caring-healing." (Watson, 2008, p.09)

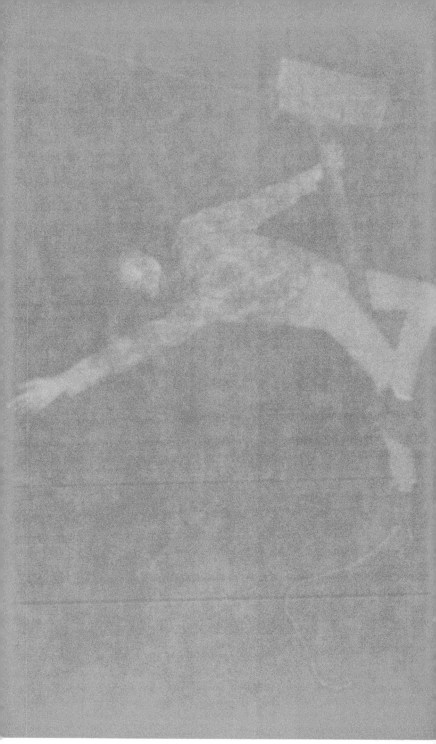

Chapter II

Times of uncertainty

Once the radiotherapy in São Paulo was over, we returned to Montevideo. Those were very difficult times with a great deal of uncertainty regarding Julieta's health. We were hoping that the treatment might work and that she would have a chance to get better.

By now, Juli was entering puberty and her longings and aspirations were focused on leading a normal teenage life like going out with her friends and engaging in activities, as well as resuming her studies and starting high school

But there was something that caused me a great deal of stress and anguish: the visits for the CT scan results. It was during these visits that we needed to face the harsh reality. Was everything going to be okay, or were we going to start all over again? After all, it was Julieta's first CT scan taken when she was only 6 years old that had revealed the complexity of the situation we were facing (even though the confirmation of the sort of tumor we were dealing with and the seriousness of the illness came later, after the biopsy).

She went through dozens of CT scans and radiographies, MRIs, bone scintigraphy's (a scan procedure to identify abnormal areas or lesions in the bones) and two PET scans (Positron Emission Tomography).

I must admit that it was these situations that really distressed me, moments that I would rather have spared myself from, but I knew I ought to be there for her and be strong for the family. To comfort and reassure Julieta who always felt protected when next to me.

Because she felt so reassured by me, Juli wouldn't let anyone else puncture her with a needle. Most of the IV lines were inserted by me, which brought additional stress to the situation because I had to make sure I did it properly, and without failing my daughter.

As a professional I acknowledge this wasn't the most appropriate thing to do, but on the other hand it was the human thing to do. The transpersonal moment had always been present with me and Julieta. Those moments were of a profound spiritual connection for both of us, which brought tranquility and reassurance to us. It was a moment of loving kindness to see my daughter going through difficult situations with confidence and optimism thanks to our beautiful father-daughter connection and the sacred art of caring.

"The sacred art of caring is an act of love, a much deeper work linked to life." (Watson, 2005, p. 64)

It is difficult to explain, it is metaphysical and subjective. Sacred art focuses on experience and ethics, intuition and intention. Feeling and sharing the care of loving kindness with others and kindness towards oneself, strengthening transpersonal relationships.

Watson's Caring Science shares the belief that in order to fully care for another person, we have to have a loving, kind, and compassionate relationship with ourselves first.

A few months after our return to Montevideo when everything seemed to be going well and we had begun to slowly resume our normal daily lives, we noticed a small deformation in her face – something was wrong.

The exams confirmed that the illness had reappeared.

The situation became impossible. The cancer was coming back earlier and earlier and more aggressively each time and we knew there were no longer any chances of a treatment. It is indescribable to capture in words the feelings I experienced during this time. I was devastated, I felt helpless, angry, and experienced moments of great sadness. This was the third recurrence, and the fourth time that the cancer had appeared.

Decision time

We had many difficult conversations with the medical teams.

Resuming the oncology treatments would only help to ease the symptoms, we already knew that there weren't any more chances of a cure. Knowing how little time she had, she would need to spend it in the hospital, most probably in isolation due to the aggressiveness of the treatment and her general state of health.

The other option was to start palliative care. Making that decision wasn't easy at all. As a parent, one always wants the best for one's children. In those moments we needed to think about what was best for her and what would make her happier.

We knew that Julieta loved being with her family, her friends, her pets, and her toys; and having the opportunity to enjoy the freedom of going to a park, or to the beach, or for a walk along the promenade. We decided to begin palliative care at home.

She lived for over a year without aggressive treatments, only with pain management.

I thought it would be appropriate here to transcribe Module 3 from my CCEP (Caritas Coach Education Program®). I was asked to reflect on my personal experience of how love and the conscious heart influenced my own care and healing and that of others, centered on the ontological heart and on the human evolutive tasks of Forgiveness, Gratitude, Surrender and Compassionate Human Service. This is what I wrote:

"It is about a profound and loving relationship between father and daughter born out of the pain and the compassion of going through the illness of my youngest daughter Julieta, who lived half of her life fighting cancer. Countless surgeries, radiotherapies and chemotherapies were part of her life. On her third recurrence, and after a ferocious fight against the cancer, we understood that it was necessary to stop fighting and surrender and accept other kinds of challenges, in this case palliative care, the outcome of which you are all familiar with…"

Surrendering and approaching Julieta's best year without surgeries and invasive procedures was the right thing. We shared happy and unforgettable moments as a family, especially she and her siblings. She was able to enjoy nature and many things that made her happy like her pets, her friends, her home. The interventions ended and the pain was managed. Julieta was free that last year, living intensely each moment of her short life.

What else can I say? It was very difficult to take this decision, to stop fighting and to surrender. Now, from a distance, I see it was the best decision. It is impossible to believe that one can manage in a situation like this; but one finally realises that there is no control over any of it.

This big life crisis brought such a transformation to myself that today I'm sharing with you this beautiful journey of a good and loving human being walking the path of my own care and caring for others in the same way.

Regarding the tasks centered on the ontological heart, Dr. Watson says that it is necessary to give a new and deeper meaning to the professional concept of self-discipline for the spiritual growth of consciousness itself.

With regards to the evolutionary human task of surrender and forgiveness, I surrendered from focusing on the story with my daughter, and the approach to life conditioned and centered on the head and controlled by the ego. "This is one of the most difficult lessons for our self-healing and re-patterning of ways of Being."(Watson, 2005, p. 118)

With regards to Forgiveness: "If one has to truly heal, one has to learn to forgive." (Watson, 2005, p. 115) In my case, I had to learn how to forgive myself and stop believing I was omnipotent.

On gratitude: "… evolution towards a higher consciousness for healing, is necessary to cultivate gratitude for life and all its blessings in the midst of pain, despair, turmoil change and unknowns." (Watson, 2005-p117)

Palliative Care

We began the palliative care period with an amazing team from the Pediatric Hospital of Uruguay, directed by Dr. Mercedes Bernarda. *The support and care this team provided not only to Julieta but also to the rest of the family meant the world to us.*

Palliative Care

There is a tendency to think that
Palliative Care is the preparation
for the end of life but we have to
understand that Palliative Care is the
beginning of a new stage where the
person needing caring for is provided
with all aspects of care: medical,
nursing, psychological and social care,
as well as holistic and spiritual care,
so he/she can face this new path with
dignity and surrounded by loving
care and joy.

Julieta was the first child in Uruguay to receive palliative care at home. This is a very special situation because until then, this kind of care was only provided in the hospital setting. However, as the Pediatric Hospital had been my place of work for over 20 years, I was able to speak with the medical team and my co-workers about the situation, asking them to allow Julieta to stay at home. They gave me their support. The palliative care team then agreed to help us take care of her at home with the collaboration of the palliative care team of the Hospital Maciel (which already had home care but only for adults). In this way, a spontaneous team was set up to carry out Julieta's care from home.

My infinite thanks to all these people from the palliative care team who made it possible for Julieta to have quality and truly heart centered care in the last stages of her life. She was never readmitted to the hospital, and everything was taken care of at home. This was also the beginning of a new era in Uruguay, because thanks to Julieta, home palliative care for children in Uruguay was pioneered!

There was one activity that played an important role for my self-care during this difficult time of my life: walking. I would put aside time in my daily routine to walk. I committed at least 30 minutes to an hour of walking. It is very important to make space, even just for a short period, to care for the carer. Walking provided me with relaxation, it helped me to pause during those distressing moments and to strengthen my spirit to be able to carry on. It helped to exercise my body and oxygenate my psyche. I'm recommending walking because that's what I did, but each person can find their own activity where they can feel centered, re-energised and to reconnect them with their true essence.

During this year and a half, Julieta had the opportunity to be free from difficult and painful treatments and to be able to fully enjoy the things she loved the most such as outdoor activities and contact with nature, spending time with family, friends, dogs and cats; all of which gave her so much joy.

I must acknowledge that these were difficult times. Physically the cancer kept growing though she was never in pain – she was very well managed by the palliative care team – and thanks to the medication she was able to do just about anything she wanted. Aesthetically, the beginning of this stage was very tough – especially for a young girl who is entering puberty – but with her strength, spirit and resilience she didn't give up! She carried on onward and upwards ...

To cover and hide the area where the tumor was, she decided to use scarves and amazingly without any trepidation she would go out. Her social life was very active. Nothing stopped her from going to places where there were many people, like shopping centers and malls, parks, the cinema, the theatre – anywhere she wanted to go.

Julieta was and is a great spiritual teacher. Her gift to us was the meaning and understanding as to why, in the face of the worst adversity, one must carry on, confront life and turn negative experiences into positive ones – our best option if we are to fully enjoy every minute of our lives.

During this time, we engaged in many activities: we climbed hills, enjoyed trips to various beaches, traveled around the country and abroad and visited parks, zoos, cities and towns.

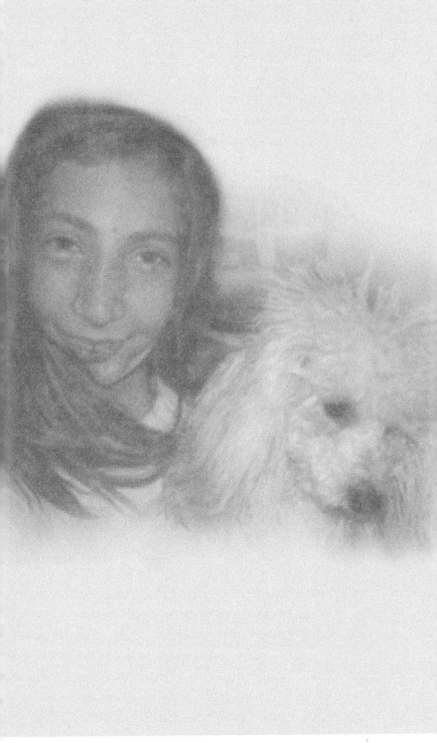

There is a trip in particular that I'd like to share: the weekend we spent at a spa in the Costa de Oro in Uruguay. This was one of Juli's last trips; she was beginning to deteriorate further physically, and the demolishing presence of cancer was becoming more obvious. Even so, Juli kept going with her great spiritual energy that mitigated those difficult moments. However, she needed more time to rest in order to recover her physical strength.

It was winter and cold, but the night was beautiful, full of stars. We were by the sea and we could see the sky lit up and the full moon. All of the family shared a barbecue and played board games and cards and later I decided to watch the beautiful sky together with Julieta and Lucia. Sharing that magnificent starry sky with my two daughters was such a special moment. We chatted for a bit about the different constellations, their shapes and names. We admired the beauty of the big moon and a completely clear sky with only the sound of the sea in the background. It was a spectacular experience that fills my heart with happiness and makes me feel proud to have had the opportunity to witness and share this with them.

When we were chatting about the constellations, we stopped at Orion, known in Latin America and Spain as 'The Three Marys.' There was a moment of deep spiritual connection and communion between us as we looked at that constellation. We said to each other that when the day comes when one of us goes, we will meet each other on that star shining in the center of the constellation we were looking up at.

Wow! The energy going through my body right now as I remember it brings tears to my eyes and gives me goosebumps. It was an unforgettable and transformative moment and since then, every time I see the starry sky, I immediately connect with my daughter and her boundless love.

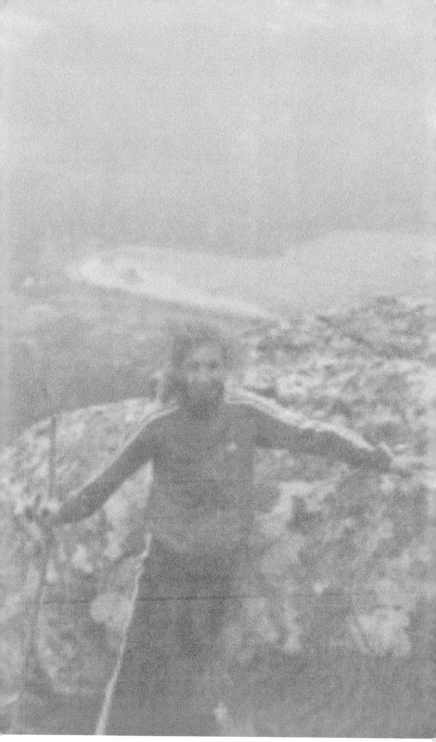

The way my parents dealt with Julieta's situation and the impact it was having on us was something that saddened and upset me during this time. I didn't have the support from them that I'd expected. They didn't know how to deal with the situation. It was so painful that it paralyzed them; they didn't have the tools to face it. They didn't know how to support me and that was terribly painful for me. I think that perhaps by just being there for me even without saying anything would have been very helpful and important for me. Nevertheless, I forgave them – and I forgave myself. As I did so, it became a very important and healing experience in order for me to be able to move on with my life.

In July we were able to organise and celebrate Juli's last birthday, she was turning 13. We had a big party with friends and family at her home and she had the opportunity to enjoy the tropical music band she loved so much who played live especially for her. She had a wonderful time. The illness was by then at a very advanced stage and her general deterioration was very noticeable. We all wanted to appear happy and in a party mood, but the bittersweet feeling was clearly palpable.

Julieta enjoyed intensely her last years of life. Being in nature was very important to her, and so during those last days we used to take her out in the car, something she would look forward to which would comfort her and re-energise her spiritually.

Juli used several complementary therapies but there was one in particular, hypnotherapy, which really helped her prepare for the moment of death. A pediatrician who specialised in hypnotherapy from the Pediatric Hospital (guided by the palliative care unit) carried out the sessions. We did several sessions at home. There was one experience where Julieta was taught how to imagine herself in a beautiful place where she could feel at ease, comfortable and at peace. If she needed to find relief from anguish or stress, she could always reflect upon this place and imagine herself there. I took part in all of the sessions and so I learned how to help Juli to induce this state of trance so she could reach that personal special place in order to soothe her during difficult times when she needed to alleviate physical or psychological discomfort.

The day of her death

We were in the middle of October 2013, and Julieta's general state of health had greatly deteriorated; we knew her departure was only a matter of hours away.

My own feelings of pain and anguish and those of my family were unbearable. We supported and comforted each other the best we could in order to cope.

And so, the day of her death arrived. It was a spring day. The day had begun with radiant sunshine. Julieta was serene and at peace with no pain thanks to the medication. We could perceive that the end was coming. Close and extended family from both sides (mine and her mum's) gathered. Friends and neighbors joined us during this heavy farewell.

In the afternoon of October 19th, 2013, Julieta died surrounded by her family. I was holding one hand and her mum was holding the other. Her siblings were next to her by her bed. Surrounded by the love of her parents and siblings, Julieta took her last breath. She departed with much peace and serenity leaving behind lessons on the importance of living life intensely with love and goodness. It is impossible to describe in words this moment of such intense and painful feelings but, above all, there was a feeling of pure love in the heart which filled the emptiness of her departure.

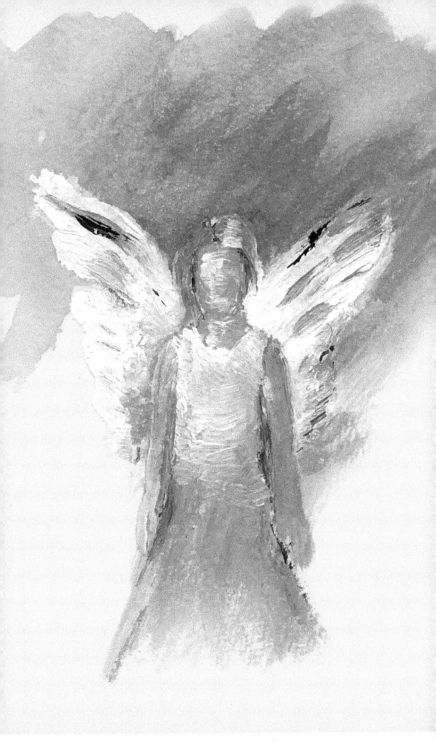

"As the sages say, without honoring death, we are not fully alive. Indeed, in the cosmic sense again, we are dying every moment, in that with each breath we experience the miracle of life itself and the precious, yet delicate, nature of how we are held in the hands of that which is greater than us. And at a deeper metaphysical or metaphorical level, or within Native American cosmology of or in any indigenous belief system, death is not the end, it is a continuation of the sacred wheel of life. And as the expression goes: Who is to say that life is not death, and death is not life?" (Watson, 2005, p. 138)

Chapter III

The denial period

For two years I was in denial, feeling unmoved and making a big effort to carry on. I was feeling like a robot – only focusing on my work, my studies, and on providing financial support for others; but failing to honor my great loss, my grief, and my need for self-care and healing.

I began a dual Master's degree in Strategic Management with a specialisation in Healthcare Organisations and I had received promotions, which created even more responsibilities in both of my jobs: as Chief of Pediatric Nursing and Specialties at the Pediatric Hospital of the Centro Hospitalario Pereira Rossell, and as Head of Department at the Universidad Católica of Uruguay.

During this period, it was also very important to me to be present and support my other two children, Enzo and Lucia. We would meet several times a week, particularly on weekends. We'd share an evening meal or barbecue and chat, or spend the day out doing various activities, or walking in nature. During this tough time, these were very special moments of connection and closeness for us. Sometimes I would meet with both Lucia and Enzo together, other times separately, but all time spent was equally important, supportive, and comforting.

For myself – I was doing next to nothing.

I was helping my children face their pain, but I wasn't facing my own … I wanted to run away from my own grief.

Impossible.

Caring for myself was set aside although I did continue to go for my walks – which was perhaps one of the only things I did for my own self-care. The walks gave me the opportunity to exercise and have some time exclusively dedicated to listening to myself in order to reflect, to remember, release tension, think and dream.

It was during the first months of 2015 when I began to face my own pain.

For several months in Montevideo I saw a professional psychologist who was a good fit for me. She helped me and made me confront my grief and pain.

During this period, I understood the need to do things for myself and to dedicate time to my self-care.

"As a beginning, we have to learn how to offer caring, love, forgiveness, compassion, and mercy to ourselves before we can offer authentic caring and love to others."

(Watson, 2008, p. 41)

Trip to Paraguay

In August of that year, I was invited to participate in a nursing conference in Paraguay. I accepted the invitation and instinctively knew it was very important to take this trip alone as a starting point for this new period, centered on my own self-care. I felt an internal force, a kind of inspiring energy that was telling me for some reason this trip was going to be very important for me.

I didn't know how to fill the big emptiness and pain I felt within myself, but at the same time I also felt an inexplicable uncontrollable force, a force that motivated me, pushing me forward, compelling me to make a big change in my life.

So, I began to plan my trip, making sure that there was going to be time for me.

I could have taken a plane and been in Asunción in less than two hours, but I didn't. I decided to drive.

Driving my car is for me a projection of my body and my spirit; I feel very comfortable driving, plus it would be the perfect connection with Julieta – connecting to my pain and her deep love. In addition, driving would allow me to get absorbed in the road trip, to enjoy the scenery and nature. So, there I went, driving my car on this long return trip of 3,000 Kilometers from Montevideo, Uruguay, to Asunción, Paraguay. My only company being my mate tea (a typical tea from Uruguay), and a little cuddly stuffed toy dog that had joined Julieta and me on many trips that we had shared. This little dog reminded me of the times we had spent together, of those beautiful moments, filled with love and care.

I began my trip in Montevideo and drove to Young in Uruguay, and then crossed over into Argentina on the International Bridge. I drove through part of northern Argentina until I arrived in Asunción. On my way back, I drove through southern Paraguay to the city of Encarnación, and then crossed over into Argentina through Posadas, continuing until Uruguayana in Brazil, entering Uruguay from Brazil, through Rivera, and finally reaching Montevideo.

I had planned my trip so I could journey through four countries and experience their very different sceneries and landscapes. I needed my own space, privacy, and time to really be in connection with my inner self, my essence and my spirit.

I experienced special moments during these long periods of driving, which provided the space and time for inner reflection. The trip was so important for my healing. It was revealing and rich with many moments and stages of the journey that have and will forever be engraved in my retina and in my heart.

Of course, there were difficult and painful times, but above all there was healing.

I cried, I laughed, I sang, I kicked, I shouted. I forgave others and I forgave myself. At times I was sad, at other times I was happy. I listened to my own voice for the first time in a long time. It was incredible. My own voice coming from the deepest part of my being, my spirit talking to me. It was amazing! I could truly feel my sadness, my anger, my rage and my guilt.

After having experienced all of these emotions, a sense of great inner peace and calm filled me completely; my heart opened. I felt a very strong connection with my spirit.

The pain of the death of a child never goes away – it will always be there – but we can learn to live with it.

This moment divided my life into "before" and "after."

After this trip, I began to walk the path of my grief in a different way. There had been a shift which led me to an expansion of my consciousness, allowing a connection with my essence and the universe.

"As one continues to cultivate a contemplative, meditative practice … one increasingly becomes connected with the transpersonal dimension."
(Watson, 1999, p. 174)

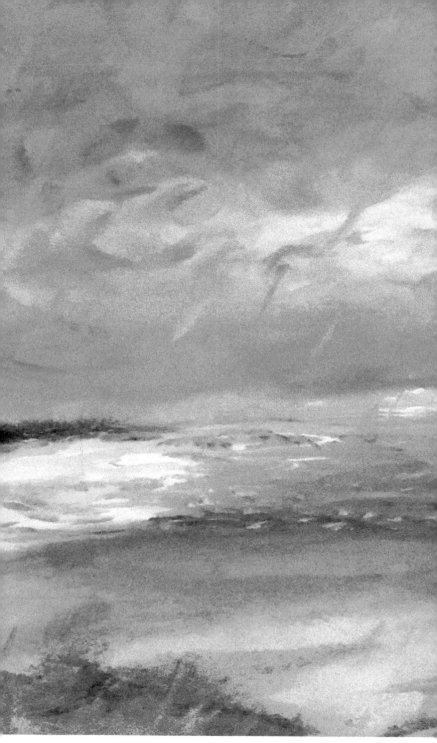

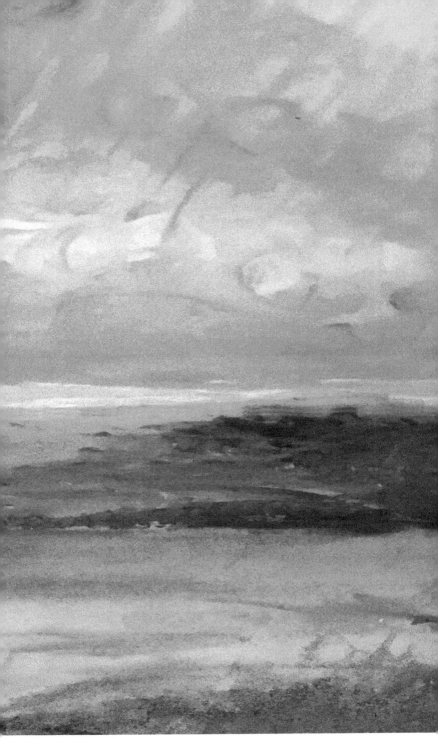

Forgiveness

I learned a lot about forgiveness during my trip to Paraguay. Having experienced all of the emotions of pain, anguish, rage and anger somehow gave way to an unspeakable inner peace and calm. I felt very strongly that I had to forgive – and to forgive my self.

And this is how my path of deepening my spiritual search began. I felt a great call to share my experiences with other people going through the same situations that I have gone through. I understood that if we really wanted to heal, we needed to learn to forgive.

Forgiveness is a hard lesson to learn and even now I still have a long way to go in this respect. Beginning to forgive myself and forgive others has transformed my life. I felt, (and still feel) that the load in my backpack had become lighter, and with this there is an embracing and liberating sense of peace.

If one commits to the spiritual path on the art of forgiveness of oneself and others, then forgiveness can be healing. I'm a great admirer of the Hawaiian philosophy for conflict resolution and spiritual healing known as 'Ho'oponopono' which is grounded in forgiveness, love and reconciliation.

I had the opportunity to put these teachings into practice to heal my relationship with my father with whom I have never had a very close relationship – quite the opposite – our relationship was distant and cold. But with time I understood that he had done all that he could for me and my sisters.

"Forgiveness of self and others seems to be a deep psychological, spiritual, if not physical-biological, task that is necessary to cleanse our psychic soul for evolving toward Love and Caring."
(Watson, 2005, p. 115)

We grew up in a household where the support came mainly from my mother. We received loving care and family values and received a good education. We grew up surrounded by a big family, with grandparents, uncles, aunties and cousins, in a neighborhood formed by a community of beautiful people that continued to conform to and strengthen those values, and that made us the good and decent people we are today.

As I was walking through this difficult but revealing period of my life and working on forgiveness, I was able to approach the relationship with my dad from a completely new perspective which came out of the maturity of life and of the experiences life had given me – that, and a great deal of love. We could talk frankly and express our feelings. This was another very special moment in my life. I forgave him and I forgave myself. This allowed the load of my life backpack to get even lighter, and I continued to fill it up with peace and love for my heart and for my soul.

Sharing these moments with my father and walking alongside each other on this path (even if only for a short time) was a gift from life. My dad died a few months later from a sudden cardiac arrest. I could deal with his departure with love and with the happiness and the joy that comes from knowing that nothing had been left unresolved between the two of us, and that I had been able to get spiritually closer to him during the last stage of his life.

Currently, I work on forgiveness every day and I'm very grateful to life and the universe for giving me opportunities to do so.

My journey through different holistic paths and disciplines

After having achieved a more spiritual connection and reconnection with my essence through the expansion of my consciousness, I began to explore several paths that would guide my search to deepen my spiritual awakening. I will list some of them and my experiences with them.

Angel reading

I began my spiritual awakening journey with an Angel Reading from a young lady of great inner peace and beauty with whom I felt a special connection.

The reading is a space where through guidance and dialogue you can listen to your Angels and receive their messages. During the reading, you share personal information around your current situation and those aspects in your life that need healing. The messages given to you are divine guidance that can help you heal and return to peace. The messages are channeled (in my case through this young lady) in an intuitive way through perceptions, feelings, visions or images which are received during this connection with the guides of light (Angels). My first and only experience was very beautiful, and I received the guidance, peace and strength I needed to carry on my spiritual journey to continue exploring other experiences which would expand my horizons and my wisdom.

I attended this session with my great friend and co-worker Adriana who lovingly calls me "younger brother." I love that, because this moment in our lives marked the beginning of spiritual paths for the both of us. Our souls twinned and we started to expand as individuals and nursing professionals committed to human caring excellence and to integrative holistic medicine.

Akashic Records

At this time, I wasn't very clear how I was going to continue my spiritual search which had begun with the deep inner peace from the Angel Reading. I felt there was more to experience, and so my search led me to Akashic Records where I found the clarity I needed to continue.

Akashic Records are a universal memory, a multidimensional space where all of the experiences of the soul are kept. Some of the messages that I received from my guides allowed me to deepen my spiritual experience through other modalities such as meditation, yoga, biodecodification therapy, Shamanic Energy, and Reiki.

Akashic Records helped me feel good. I found lightness and guidance and a place of deep connection with my spirit. I have received several Akashic Records readings and later, I trained at the Holistic Centre in Montevideo, in order to deepen my knowledge about it.

Meditation

Meditation was for me, one of the best disciplines where I find calmness, to quiet my mind, to listen to my heart, and to be more in touch with my soul.

I started this path thanks to the excellent guidance of the Gendai Integral Therapist Center of Montevideo, and through attending several retreats and meditative practice sessions, surrounded by nature.

Through practice, I began to understand how important something as simple as breathing is in order to have a good meditative technique, but also to help us pause, to have a moment to center ourselves during difficult situations, in times of stress, or simply to start the working day and face day to day situations and activities.

"We can start a simple process and practice of Centering in the moment, by a simple pause, 'breathing', and emptying out. We learn how to connect with, learn how to hold that still point, how to hold the void, that miracle point between
the in breath and the
out breath."
(Watson, 2008, p. 54)

"Within the practice of 'Caritas Nursing', which embraces such meditative practices of equanimity and loving-kindness toward oneself and other, we have advantages in our daily life. Our mindful, caring presence affects others; it increases our level of energy and creativity for our work without

wasting or dribbling
away our life energy
life force; it helps us
to observe the work
with more clarity and
discernment without
reacting inappropriately.
It helps us to
Be Present."
(Watson, 2008, p. 54)

Yoga

In yoga I found a discipline that gives me special moments of harmony and inner peace in close contact with my physical body, achieving a balanced mind and spiritual connection and integrating the three planes of existence.

Biodecodification Therapy

My experience with the technique of family tree Biodecodification Therapy helped me face and understand several inherited family situations. I did it with a person who was very well suited to the task, and who guided and supported me in dealing with many situations (health related issues in particular).

Native Latin American Spiritual Traditions

I engaged in several activities and ceremonies with Medicine Men and Women belonging to the group 'Camino de los Hijos de la Tierra' (The Path of the Children of Earth) in Uruguay. The aim of this group is to organise cultural, educational and spiritual activities in order to raise awareness, retrieve and preserve the way of life and the traditions of Native Latin American Populations.

According to this tradition, the spirit (or God) is one unique being called "Great Spirit" which sustains all forms of life, including humans and the rest of creation.

I remember with great joy and love one weekend retreat deep within nature (inland in Uruguay) where I shared unforgettable moments with a group of beautiful people. A number of sacred medicine ceremonies were performed, during which ancient native spiritual wisdom was shared. This was followed by long reflective group discussions (sitting in a circle) and moments of deep personal inner connection. We sang songs and offered prayers and expressions of gratitude. The ceremony of Temazcal (sweat lodge ceremony) was very beautiful and gave me a powerful connection with my essence and my spirit forging my spiritual path.

Out of all my experiences with the different sacred medicines there was one that made me face my deepest fears, the Ayahuasca (ancient plant medicine). The effect it had on me was very special. I felt I had died to be reborn. I experienced a mixture of very intense and diverse feelings and I let myself go, guided by my intuition and my heart without creating any resistance. I completely surrendered to the process, let go and thus discovered and felt a whole kaleidoscope of deep feelings and emotions. Once the experience was over, I felt surrounded by great calmness and an immense peace. My backpack was even lighter. My heart and my body were embraced by love and goodness. My mind had witnessed a beautiful experience without any intervention from the logical mind.

Reiki

One of the disciplines I fell in love with was Reiki. I feel a very special connection when I become a channel of the universal energy that enables me to help to heal myself and others. It has many similarities with my nursing profession in the sense of helping to heal and applying healing for the benefit of oneself and/or others.

This was the last modality I trained for in Uruguay, and today I practice it and continue my training. It makes me feel well and happy to do so. I have been able to increase my channel with the universe, especially when I have the chance to visit energetic places and particularly when I meditate.

All of these disciplines, groups, and techniques helped my healing, my connection, my inner growth and my spiritual expansion.

For me everything is interconnected. We are all one!

Emotional Detachment

Several times in my life I have taken another path, turned around and pulled away from a loved one, but there are two occasions in particular which really affected me and made me reflect on emotional detachment – on how painful it is and how much one needs to fight against the ego to leave this comfort zone.

On both occasions, I still feel a great deal of love for these people, but this love was transformed/altered, and my own transformation became a priority when I began to feel an incredible moving force inside myself telling me to carry on with my own path. During those times, the path split into two and I decided to walk a solo path. It could sound selfish but sometimes it is necessary. This is the way I feel, and it is part of the process of personal inner growth.

Love for oneself comes first – even if in this instance it was really difficult to love myself – but I have felt this self-love recently and it is immensely beautiful and has connected me with my essence.

I think there are times in life when we need to put some distance in place in order to see things with a different perspective and, if we are in a space of loving pain, this can often lead to a reinvention of the self.

Losses can become opportunities, to get close to oneself and others in different situations so that we can feel empowered and take the right road that leads to self-transformation.

Often, the person who stays blames the person who has left,

and this can be lived as a burden. In these times it was necessary for me to cultivate self-compassion and determination in order to carry on moving forward.

I think it´s important to express, to forgive oneself, and to forgive others. It is one of the best ways to free us from guilt, even if it is painful.

Now I apply all of these forms of knowledge to myself and I'm aware of how necessary self-care of the body, mind, soul, and the whole of me; are in life.

As Jean Watson says, the sacred art of Caring is an act of love. It focuses on experience and ethics, intuition and intention. Feeling and sharing the act of loving kindness with others and kindness towards oneself, strengthens care within transpersonal relationships.

Spiritual connection with family

During this very special period of my life I managed to connect with and get spiritually closer to my sister Cecilia. Our relationship had always been relatively close … but not very close; perhaps life and its circumstances made it this way. But it was during this time of increasing spiritual awakening that I felt compelled to get closer to her. And this happened through the search for spirituality.

It was after I shared one of my Akashic Record reading sessions with her that she decided to start exploring the world of spiritual connection. Now we share the same language and the same philosophy. She has trained as a yoga instructor and in Reiki and Bach Flower Remedies. She currently has her own holistic center. I'm so happy and joyful about this new stage of our brother-sister relationship.

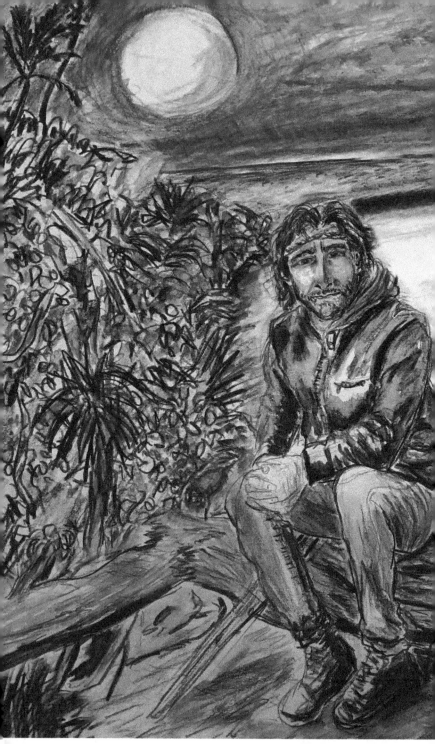

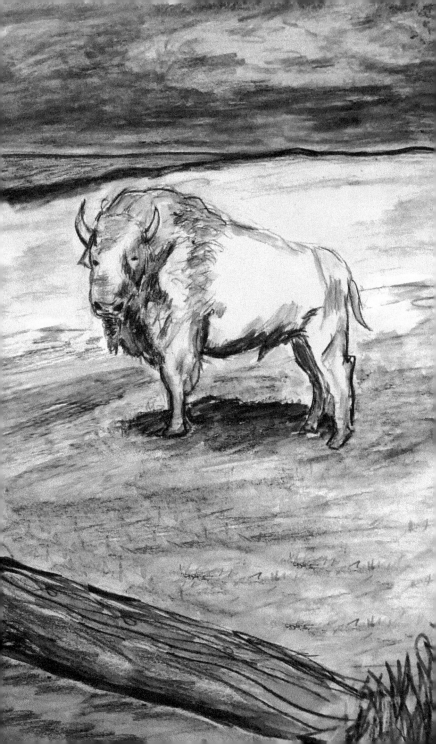

Chapter IV

My New Path

During this period, I felt very strongly that I needed to make real changes in my life, so this is where I put my focus and intention, and I can say I am grateful to have done so!

A new awakening and consciousness of the self has begun. I went from profound loss, to the need to heal, through to the different spiritual disciplines; leading me to further deepen my personal search. I continue my search for myself, paying attention to my intuition to shift to an open heart, my introspection, and my connection to the universe.

In November 2017, I attended a nursing conference on Human Caring in Chile where I had the wonderful opportunity to hear for the first time the world-renowned nurse theorist and philosopher Dr. Jean Watson. Years ago, during Nursing school, I remember in my Epistemology class we studied nurse theorists, and Dr. Jean Watson was without a doubt the most important one.

As I shared time with co-workers and friends from all over the world at the conference, I began to better understand Caring Science theory. Within myself, I noticed a feeling of fulfillment and well-being. For me, this theory was the perfect complement to the profession I love – nursing, and to all of the many disciplines related to health and holistic care.

On the plane back home, I spent time reflecting on the conference I had just experienced, and said to myself, "This is my new path, my new life." My heart was telling me I should move ahead. This gave me a sense of confidence and peace that filled my soul, a feeling so strong I decided to take a step forward to make it happen.

This meant I would need to leave many things behind, such as my job and my professional career of more than 28 years in the National Health Service Administration in Uruguay. This was a secure and stable job funded by the Government. My position during the previous two years had been as a Deputy Director of Medical Occupational and Psychosocial Rehabilitation in a large psychiatric hospital in Montevideo.

Only two months had passed since my first contact with Caring Science when I set off to the USA and began my new life. I had to train and learn more. I started my training through the Watson Caring Science Institute (WCSI) on their Caritas Coach Education Program® (CCEP) in Colorado. This training has the endorsement of the American Holistic Nurses Association.

And since then, I've been walking the path of the science of loving-kindness. I'm currently a Doctoral Scholar in Caring Science working with Dr. Watson at the Watson Caring Science Institute, and it is my intention to continue on this path so I can delve into Caring Science and loving-kindness in order to be able to share this way of life, particularly in Latin America.

During this time, I had to address a difficult barrier. CCEP is taught in English and so, while I was training, I also had to face the study of the English language. Learning English was, and still is, a massive personal challenge. I had only basic English language understanding acquired mainly in high school, but in reality, it feels like I am starting from scratch, and when one has reached a certain age, the situation is ever more challenging! I committed and still commit many hours of study daily in order to improve my second language.

Learning English took me to England. At the time, I was beginning a new and beautiful relationship with my partner, and now wife, Julie, a very special person full of love, goodness, light, and who possesses a very special commitment to help others. She gave me the support and the confidence to move forward on my new path, especially in England.

It is always difficult to start a new life in a foreign country, particularly when language and cultural differences are vast and even more so in my case, because I was splitting my time between the USA and England (by the way, the only thing they have in common is the language!). In the USA, I shared time with my family who live in Florida which made me feel supported: my sister Elizabeth, my brother-in-law, my nephews and nieces, and my mother who had moved to my sister's place after my father's death. My sister was always there to support me and to help me as much as she could. Having family in a new country is a big advantage that really makes a difference.

Caritas Coach Education Program

What is a Caritas Coach®?

"The Caritas Coach Education Program (CCEP) is based on Dr. Jean Watson's renowned theory of human Caring Science. It is a unique, six-month professional development program which incorporates interactive online instruction, virtual small group intensives, and an assigned Caritas Coach faculty mentor.

Through dynamic inquiry and collaborative, compassionate dialogue, participants explore Caritas consciousness and ways of knowing-being-doing-becoming, which prepare the student to transform their personal and professional life practice toward deeper meaning, purpose, dignity and wholeness. As a Caritas Coach, participants return to their work setting and personal life with new insight, wisdom, and skills to give voice as "living caritas": better able to translate and "live out" the theory and philosophy of human caring-healing, in service for deep system transformation.

The outcome sought will be to transform the professional caring nurse/health care provider into an inspired leader – a Caritas Coach".

(www.watsoncaringscience.org/caritas-coach-education-program-ccep).

The training consists of two weekend on-site seminars, (which in my case took place in Boulder and Denver, Colorado). One is at the beginning of the program and the second is at the end of the training. Graduation takes place during the last weekend, with presentation of a final project by each participant, and a graduation ceremony conducted by Dr Watson.

I started the course feeling very happy. I shared the weekend with a group of amazing people committed to the study and the reflection on Caring Science, and my classmates were open to sharing their experiences about life and about the act of caring. This first contact and all that followed during the seminars and workshops was very enlightening for me, both personally and professionally.

One of the first assignments I was asked to carry out was to share with the group a personal reflection on what had led me to Caring Science. I briefly elaborated on what I had lived through with Julieta, my journey after her death, my feelings and my commitment to deepening my spiritual path.

The reaction to my reflection from Jan Anderson, CCEP Program Director, was as follows:

"Dearest Héctor,
To be so close to suffering affects us at the soul level – our heart and soul are forever changed – either positively – or not. Your ability to translate the experience you shared with your daughter through all the treatments, pain, joy and suffering into a more expanded perspective of what caring and healing mean not just for individuals and families, but for communities, countries and the world, is a healing as well. Jean believes that what we do as nurses is sacred and that when we begin to more fully realise that sacredness of all that we do, say, think, intend ... can make a difference, then we can become more aware and conscious of ourselves and make more biogenic choices, you have done this by honoring your daughter and all you both have experienced into something more far reaching."

This was a great start on my path to dive deeper into Caring Science. Jan's comments strengthened my sense of belonging and the way I felt about continuing to walk on this path, guided by my heart and my soul.

What being a Caritas Coach means to me

For me, Caritas is the beginning of a profound journey of communion with my most divine essence, to feel empowered through different spiritual disciplines and experiences which are helping me to grow personally, professionally, and collectively through sharing with others.

Deepening the theory of human caring allows me to be a conduit of Caritas teachings, ethics, and values. This allows me to share them with a variety of people: with my colleagues who are often completely immersed in the routine of their duties; with students – who are the future of nursing; and with other health professionals. My aim is to convey this theory so the health paradigm can be changed in every corner of Latin America.

Caritas offers the opportunity to study and to take care of all the facets of our being so we can provide integral and holistic care to others whilst treating every person with respect and dignity.

Dr. Watson says Love is the highest level of consciousness and the greatest healer; this creates an opening where we can practice loving-kindness towards oneself and others, clearing the way for miracles.

Caring for others with the intention to heal and transfer that energy with human consciousness and presence.

Dr. Watsons's 10 Caritas Processes® are our guiding light in the act of caring.

They include the importance of the transpersonal caring relationship which is to get to the essence of another person, to connect so we can offer the care needed, paying special attention to the spiritual dimension as well.

A conscious act of caring is opening to another person and adjusting to the new, considering all the many healing modalities, opening to different ways and styles of healing, whatever they might be, believing, encouraging, supporting and paying enough attention to the caring relationship with oneself and others, guided by ethical, moral and philosophical values.

For me, deepening my spiritual path alongside this most beautiful profession of nursing is why I am here. Acquiring new knowledge and delving into the theory of human caring, being able to live out, share and multiply this theory is what I am.

10 CARITAS PROCESSES ®

1. Sustaining humanistic-altruistic values by practice of loving–kindness, compassion and equanimity with self/others.

2. Being authentically present, enabling faith/hope/belief system; honoring subjective inner, life-world of self/others.

3. Being sensitive to self and others by cultivating own spiritual practices; beyond ego-self to transpersonal presence.

4. Developing and sustaining loving, trusting-caring relationships.

5. Allowing for expression of positive and negative feelings - authentically listening to another person's story.

6. Creatively problem-solving, 'solution-seeking' through caring process; full use of self and artistry of caring-healing practices via use of all ways of knowing/being/doing/becoming.

7. Engaging in transpersonal teaching and learning within context of caring relationship; staying within others' frame of reference-shift toward coaching model for expanded health/wellness.

8. Creating a healing environment at all levels; subtle environment for energetic authentic caring presence.

9. Reverentially assisting with basic needs as sacred acts, touching mindbodyspirit of others; sustaining human dignity.

10. Opening to spiritual, mystery, unknowns – allowing for miracles (Watson 2008).

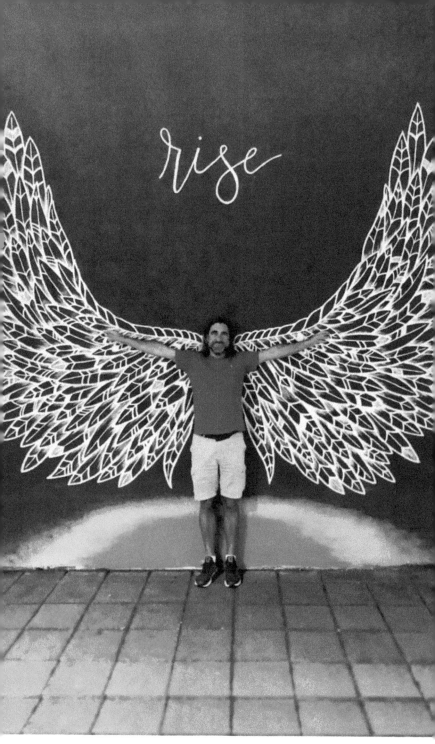

Caritas Coach Declaration:

I, Héctor, as a nurse and as a person, commit to consciously care for myself and others so that I can continue to heal and evolve, to further deepen my Caritas spiritual and empirical path in order to share this way of being/becoming and contribute to values for the sake of a better world/planet.

"A Centering exercise is one way to enter into, prepare for, and begin a more formal cultivation of the practice of Loving-Kindness and Equanimity as professional Caritas Consciousness." (Watson, 2008, p. 51).

Centering Practices

It is ideal to start the day with a centering exercise which can be done during difficult and stressful times as a way to pause and center so that we can regain calmness, peace, tranquillity, and the stillness needed to carry on, trying to let go of what's troubling us.

I find meditation to be a centering practice. Meditation can be done by anyone and in any way they feel most comfortable. There are many techniques available to choose from.

The most important thing for me is to start by centering my attention on the breath, taking my time and focusing on deep and sustainied inhales and exhales.

As Jean Watson says: "As one continues to cultivate a contemplative, meditative practice ... one becomes connected with the transpersonal dimension of life." (Watson, 1999, p. 174)

Moments of Meditation

During meditation, I feel very peaceful and still, and I can quickly go to a place within, a very special place that I can only access through this practice. It is a place of connection with the universe, a place where my mind can travel and find comfort in the surroundings. It is a place where I feel an expansion of my consciousness.

When I go deep into meditation, scents become very vivid, a mixture of jungle and sea with wildflowers and spring perfumes with an amazing and inexplicable sweetness. I can see, touch, feel and interact with my surroundings. It is incredibly beautiful but has some details that make it out of this world …

Let me describe it.

It is an incredible big woodland. On one side there is the immensity of a tranquil sea with beautiful beaches and people interacting with each other, radiating a lot of light. On the other side is the beautiful woodland that, even if enormous in size, gives me a great sense of peace. The sky is blue changing into different shades of ochres around the edges. The sun is immensely big but has no movement. I always see it in the same place and strangely, I can see on the other side of the sun two moons, one full and the other crescent shaped.

I always go on the same path to get to this place. From the path I can enjoy views of the sea on one side and views of the woodland on the other. It is a path with long pastures molded by the soft breeze. As I approach it, there is an increasing sense of tranquility and complete inner peace and love that fills my soul and the whole of my body. It is immensely beautiful. I can sense and see a sort of energy or white light surrounding me.

This path always takes me to a big tree with a beautiful treehouse high up, rustic but comfortable where I feel totally at home. I can see and taste delicious fruits that are of unusual shapes and colors.

Beyond the tree, there is direct access to the beach. On several occasions I have conversed and had physical contact with the inhabitants of this place, I know many of them. Julieta is there, she is an ascended soul.

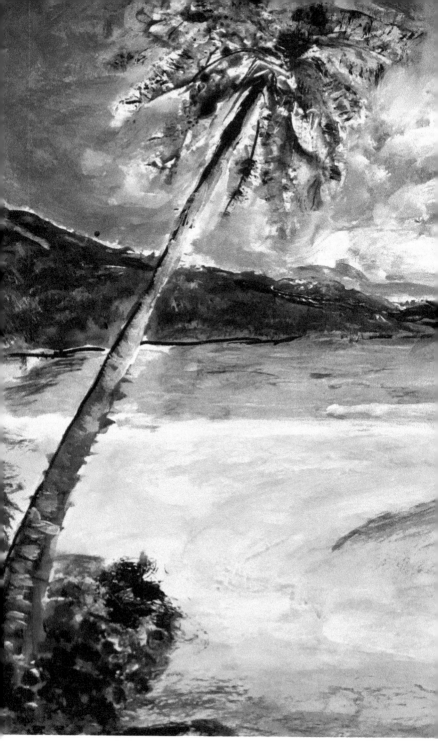

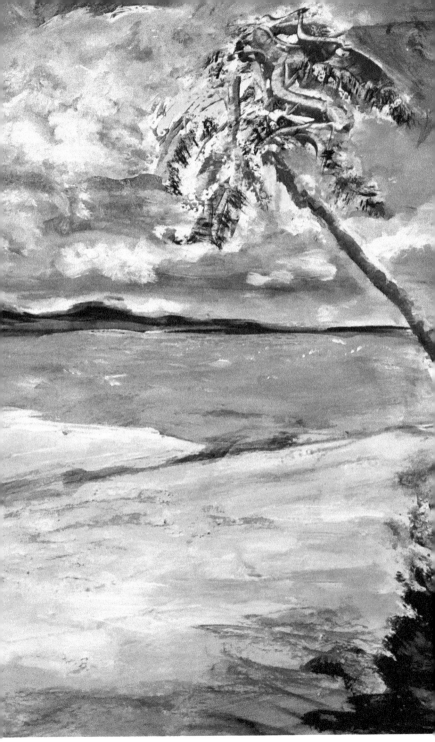

Meditation Exercise

Here is a meditation exercise I learned during my Caritas
Coach Program. I have created this as an online
meditation in Spanish which you can listen to here:
https://vimeo.com/269376189

Hand Meditation
From *Celtic Meditations* by Edward J. Farrell

Assume the same posture as with other meditations …
eyes closed, hands open and resting, palms up in your lap.

Tune into your breath. Relax any tension points,
go into your center.

Become aware of the air at your fingertips, between your fingers and
on the palms of your hands.

Experience the fullness, strength and maturity of your hands.

Think of your hands.

Think of the most unforgettable hands you have ever known,
the hands of your father, your mother, your grandparents.

Remember the oldest hands that have rested in your hands.

Think of the hands of a new-born child, your nephew, your niece, or
your own child and the incredible beauty, perfection
and delicacy in the hands of a child. Once upon a time
your hands were that same size.

Think of all that your hands have done since then.
Almost all that you have learned has been through your hands …
turning yourself over, crawling and creeping, walking and balancing
yourself, learning to hold something for the first time, feeding
yourself, washing and bathing, dressing yourself.

At one time your greatest accomplishment was tying
your shoes.

Think of all the learning your hands have done and how many activities they have mastered, the things they have made, remember the day you learned to write your own name.

Our hands were not just for ourselves but also for others. How often they were given to help another.

Remember all the kinds of work they have done, the tiredness and aching they have known, the cold and the heat, the soreness and the bruises, remember the tears they have wiped away, our own or another's, the blood they have bled, the healing they have experienced.

How much hurt, anger or even frustration they have given.

How often they have folded in prayer: a sign of both their powerlessness and of their power.

Our father and mother guided these hands in a great symbolic language ... the sign of the cross, the striking of our breast, the handshake, the wave of the hand in hello and goodbye.

There is a mystery that we discover in the hand of a woman or the hand of a man that we love.

There are the hands of a doctor, a nurse, an artist, a conductor, and a priest, hands that you can never forget.

Now raise your right hand slowly and gently place it over your heart.

Press more firmly for a moment until your hand picks up the beat of your heart, that most mysterious of all human sounds, one's own heartbeat, a rhythm learned in the womb from the heartbeat of one's mother.

Press more firmly for a moment and then release your hand and hold it just a fraction from your clothing. Experience the warmth between your hand and your heart.

Now lower your hand to your lap very carefully as if it is carrying your heart, for it does.

When you extend your hand to another it's not just bone and skin, it's your heart.

A handshake is the real heart transplant.

Think of all the hands that have left their imprint on you. Fingerprints and handprints are heart prints that can never be erased.

The hand has its own memory. Think of all the people who bear your heart print, they are indelible and will last forever ...

Caring for the carer: a loving, kind and compassionate relationship with ourselves

I totally agree with the Caring Science belief that reflects on the following: we cannot fully care for others if we don't start with our own care first, deepening and strengthening the relationship with ourselves with compassion, kindness and love.

However, it is really hard to comprehend and digest what this means! I can say in all honesty that I have found it really difficult...

I have always had the conviction that we must first help others, doing a good deed every day to help one's neighbor – and this is a good thing! I had it branded in me with fire since I was a child from my time with the Scouts. Those were beautiful times of learning and personal growth. My experience in the Scouts actually led me to nursing – and I love my profession. But I must admit that for many years, I had the idea that others always came first, and I can't remember if there was ever a moment for me; it was always we...

Now, older and with a backpack of important life experiences behind me, I now see and feel that self-care and love towards oneself is necessary if we are to offer compassionate love, help and care to others.

"The need for affiliation is a universal human need and forms the core of humanism."
(Watson, 2008, p. 185)

The transpersonal model

As we begin to deepen the transpersonal model of caring, curing and healing, we begin with our own healing, curing and caring in order to be able to help others.

I try to keep a daily conscious practice through meditation, relaxation and Reiki, so that I can utilise my transpersonal self and get in touch with my essence. I feel that this connection is very powerful and fills me with peace, harmony and loving-kindness.

A while back I experienced a very beautiful meditation in a very energetic place in the north of France. I was surrounded by big pine trees and a leafy wood next to a stream that harmonised the moment with its song. A warm summer breeze caressed my body and a beautiful and powerful sun energized my experience, enveloped by sweet birdsongs and the fluttering of many colorful butterflies. In this setting and in this beautiful moment I began my meditation which took me on a journey of connection with my essence and my origin. It made me feel so good and was so powerful that it expanded my consciousness and made me feel aligned and connected with the Universe.

"As one awakens to the need to cultivate a contemplative, centering practice for self, then one becomes more aware of what might be meant by the concept of authentic presence, holding an intentional caring consciousness and a professional reflective practice. One then becomes more aware of the need for ongoing spiritual, ontological development, if one is to engage in caring-healing work. This pursuit of spiritual practice then becomes the ground of our being, and the ground of any professional caring-healing practices." (Watson, 1999, p. 175)

Since I have become a Caritas Coach, I have acquired many strategies to approach a relationship with another person, both in health and in illness. Most importantly, I have learned to see the essence of the other person, and to connect at a deeper and deeper level, creating authentic connection. When we connect at the soul level it creates an overwhelming and beautiful experience filling both me and the other person with energy and loving-kindness which creates a unique, truthful and honest channel of communication resulting in loving care. At the end of this wonderful process, both people receive healing. To communicate from a space of love is so important and directs us to self-reflection and right relation with self/other/universe/planet.

"Within the context of a
caring-healing relationship,
the Caring Science model posits
an energetic nature for Caritas
Consciousness: that caring
consciousness emanates an energy
that radiates from one party to
the other. It alters the field in the
moment, helping patients
access their inner healing potential.
This healing potential is a natural
process that has to do with
being-in-right-relation."
(Quinn, 1989 in Watson, 2008, p. 77)

"Transpersonal caring is life-giving and life-receiving, making the connection between caring/Caritas and Love, allowing for an evolution of consciousness. Caritas Consciousness and a *caring moment* are transpersonal, beyond the ego of either; they constitute an eternal now."
(Watson, 2018, p. 51)

The importance of listening

Ever since I was a child, I'm certain that I developed a gift: the art of listening. I begin the conversation by listening, giving the other person as much time as they need in order to communicate. I speak only when necessary and maintain empathy and sensitivity regardless of peoples' needs and situations. I have applied this quality that defines me as a person in my work (I have had many jobs and responsibilities in NGOs, universities and hospital settings), and have always had a very positive response from others.

My gift of listening to others is the first thing I give in my role as a Caritas Coach.

" The act of listening provides another example of how to cultivate Caring Science pedagogy by living one's caritas literacy through the implementation of the 10 Caritas Processes." (Horton-Deutsch & Anderson, 2018, p. 51)

Time for loving and caring

During this recent period of my life, I have cared for, and helped to support my mother to confront the reality of living with cancer. Once again, this dreaded illness was back in my life – first with my daughter and now with my mother.

However, now I was in a different place in my life's journey. I was walking the path of Caring Science and could see health and illness from a different paradigm and also through my past experience with this disease and with healing (not to be confused with recovery). This made it possible for me to have strengthened resilience and put all of my intention towards healing my mother. Healing that was beyond the cure of cancer; it was about healing my mother as a person so she could have the endurance to face the changes in her situation, and to transcend and expand her consciousness.

As part of her medical treatment, she had to face one surgery to remove the tumor as well as chemotherapy and sessions of radiotherapy. She was living in the USA at the time and was in the care of my sister Elizabeth.

One would have thought that, being physically so far away from my mum living in England, I wouldn't be able to offer her any support or healing. But quite the opposite was true. My mother received and responded to my care through distant Reiki treatments and long motivational chats that transformed her pragmatic view of the world. She began to relax into a feeling of connection with her inner self and her essence that allowed her to approach this difficult time with a great deal of positivity.

When we are truly in alignment, we have the ability to care for and heal ourselves/other in the best possible way.

During one of my visits, my mother met Julie, my partner, and despite the language barrier they had a very special connection. It was incredible to see them interact and communicate. We stayed with her and took her to the chemotherapy sessions and imaging appointments. It was during this time when we told her that Julie and I were going to formalise our relationship and the wedding was going to be in the USA, near her, in a few months. This was an excellent motivation for her. She found ways to keep busy with the wedding preparations. This was important because one of the recent tests showed a metastasis. This was just when the treatment was about to finish, and she was convinced that she had overcome the worst.

We knew the prognosis wasn't good.

The wedding was a very special time in my life because I was beginning a new period full of love and dreams with Julie, but yet there was a bittersweet taste because of my mother's situation. However, the love synergy that surrounded the wedding helped all of us to share incredible moments of great happiness. The whole family from Uruguay, England, and the USA, gathered in Florida. The ceremony was very moving, intimate and spiritual. My mother attended both the ceremony and the party that followed. She was full of energy and happiness, and her happiness was her gift to us.

Six days after the wedding, my mum died. She left in peace and surrounded by her family.

Strengthening my new path

During this new period of my life, it made me very happy to be elected Adjunct Faculty Associate of the Watson Caring Science Institute. I'm deeply grateful to Jean Watson for giving me the opportunity and honor to be part of the Caritas family as an associate teacher. It is a personal goal and a challenge because I now have the honor of conveying and sharing Caring Science, especially in Latin America.

After the wedding, I graduated as a Caritas Coach and wrote and presented one of my first papers in English (which added an extra ingredient of stress). I felt very comfortable and supported while sharing my final project with the Caritas community.

I was also introduced to Tibetan singing bowls (metal bowls) that have a beautiful sound calibrated to certain energetic frequencies and are used especially during meditation and centering practices.

In England, I was introduced to the labyrinth meditative walk. A spiritual tool, a different kind of mediation experienced by walking around a labyrinth with harmony and stillness. By practicing it, I have felt a great sense of connection and wellbeing.

I also had the opportunity to spend beautiful moments presenting my work in Caring Science at many conferences and events around the world. In the process I have been introduced to communities, cities, countries, and cultures; thus, enriching my cultural backpack and personal experiences.

During these trips, I made sure I could visit nearby places

that were spiritually relevant to me. Over the past year, I visited the following places: Jordan's Desert Valley of the Moon (Wadi Rum) and Petra, The Holy Land of Jerusalem, the Pyramids of Giza and the Valley of the Kings, Karnak Temple in Luxor, Egypt, The Rocky Mountains in Colorado, Chichén Itzá Pyramid in Mexico, Stonehenge, and the ancient Cerne Abbas Giant in England and swimming in a cenote in Mexico.

All these places contribute to the expansion of my spiritual connection channel as well as my consciousness. I'm very grateful for these experiences.

The Congress in Uruguay

As I write this book, my goal – to share Caring Science theory with others – is becoming a reality. I will have the honor of working with my colleagues in Latin America on a visionary global human caring conference for health professionals and (most importantly) for nursing students – our future. For me this represents the result of the deep transformational work I have been focusing on.

With the universe as my guide, I act as a funnel to impart love, caring and a contribution to the world through this conference.

We are organising the 2nd Latin American Global Human Caring Conference in Montevideo, Uruguay, in collaboration with the Universidad de la República and the Universidad Católica of Uruguay. This event will gather regional leaders with expertise in human caring, with nurses and other health professionals. I feel an indescribable excitement. It will be an honor to have Dr. Jean Watson in my country giving Uruguayan nurses the opportunity to have close contact with an international theorist!

Invitation

In my life, I have been through situations of great anguish and pain, the sort of experiences that shake you and force you to see things in a different way. There is a time to stop. It forces you to reflect and to the search within yourself for the possibility of new realities and perspectives. In my case it allowed me to connect with my soul, with my essence and the universe.

But I feel that this search has only started. There is a lot to achieve, to learn, digest, and to connect with. With hindsight, I can say in all honesty that I have had loads of beautiful and positive life experiences and moments of happiness that I lived intensely.

Even in times of despair, pain and anguish, it is possible to feel love, a love that is very difficult to describe and that is beyond everything: immeasurable. Even in the direst of situations one can live moments of happiness.

Today I feel whole.

I feel my heart open.

With great happiness and rejoicing I'm living a time of learning and personal growth, sharing this new lifestyle, trying to be a better person every day, giving back to the Caritas community and to the world.

I follow my life path, I try to live every day guided by my feelings, my heart and my soul and to pursue a greater connection with my essence and with the universe.

As I continue on my path, I also carry with me what was. But I do not dwell there.

I don't live in the past, but I wouldn't want it to be different either. I have let go of the "What if…" and "If I only…".

My life experience is unique, (as is everyone else's) and, like everyone, life guides me towards the unknown and towards the love in my heart. Life is difficult and uncertain, but as human beings, we are wired to carry on and live the best we can. It is true that I'm grateful for all of it. Darkness and light have given me the wisdom and vision to live with compassion and love. This reminds me of the ancient Ho'oponopono Hawaiian mantra: "I'm sorry, please forgive me, thank you, I love you."

I invite the reader to consider my journey as a touchstone. I am you; you are me. We are all one, connected by the energetic field of Love. May my story be a catalyst so that others can share their truth. My path is open towards the future and I invite you to join me on this journey. Caring Science must travel through many voices and be experienced by many people in order to honor our covenant with humanity. Caring for ourselves so we can care for one another and, ultimately, for Mother Earth.

References

Farrel, E.J. (1976) *Celtic Meditations.* USA: Dimension
    Books.

Horton-Deutsch, S. & Anderson, J. (2018). *Caritas coaching,*
    A journey toward transpersonal caring for informed
    moral action in healthcare. Indianapolis, IN: Sigma
    Theta Tau International.

Watson, J. (1999). *Postmodern nursing and beyond.* London:
    Churchill Livingstone.

Watson, J. (2005). *Caring science as sacred science.*
    Philadelphia, PA: FA Davis.

Watson, J. (2008). *Nursing: The philosophy and science of*
    caring. (Rev.ed.) Boulder, CO: University Press
    of Colorado.

Watson, J. (2018). *Unitary caring science, The philosophy*
    and praxis of nursing.
    Louisville, CO: University Press of Colorado.

Other Resources

Camino de los hijos de la tierra:
   http://www.caminodeloshijosdelatierra.org
   /13862/Inicio

Caritas Coach Education Program: https://www.
   watsoncaringscience.org/caritas-coach-education-
   program-ccep

Centro Hospitalario Pereira Rossell (CHPR): http://www.
   pereirarossell.gub.uy/

Fundación Peluffo Giguens: http://www.fpg.com.uy/

GENDAI: https://www.centrogendai.com/

Give Kids The World Village: https://www.gktw.org/

Hand meditation: https://vimeo.com/269376189

Héctor Rosso: https://www.hectorrosso.com/

Ho'oponopono: https://en.wikipedia.org/wiki/
    Ho%CA%BBoponopono

Hospital Das Clínicas: http://www.hc.fm.usp.br/

Hospital Sirio Libanes: https://www.hospitalsiriolibanes.org.
    br/unidade-sao-paulo/Paginas/default.aspx

Make-A-Wish® Brasil: http://makeawish.org.br

Watson Caring Science Institute: https://www.
    watsoncaringscience.org/

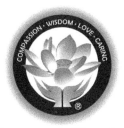

Watson Caring Science Institute

About Watson Caring Science Institute

Watson Caring Science Institute is an international non-profit 501C(3) organisation that advances the unitary philosophies, theories and practices of 'Caring Science', developed by Dr. Jean Watson. Caring Science is a transdisciplinary approach that incorporates the art and science of nursing and includes concepts from the fields of philosophy, ethics, ecology and mind-body-spirit medicine.

There are an estimated 400 hospitals throughout the USA, in which their professional practice model is based upon Watson's philosophy and theory of human caring science. The institute has trained over 500 Caritas Coaches® globally to translate caring science theory into concrete human-to-human practices that help to repattern the culture of healthcare, whereby the practitioners 'live out' the theory in their professional and personal lives.

Focusing on research, education, practice, and leadership, Watson Caring Science Institute aims to deepen the development and understanding of Caring Science and Caritas Practices®, to dramatically transform patient/family experiences of caring and healing in schools, hospitals, the wider community and our planet.

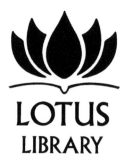

LOTUS
LIBRARY

About Lotus Library

Lotus Library is a publication imprint of Watson Caring Science Institute. Following from the philosophy of Caring Science, Lotus Library aims to encompass and showcase a humanitarian, human science orientation to human caring processes, phenomena and experiences. Our mission is rooted in compassionate care and healing of the mind-body-spirit as one. Our publications exemplify a transdisciplinary approach to sustaining caring/healing as a global covenant with humanity/Mother Earth. Lotus Library provides a forum for nurses and others to give voice to phenomena which otherwise may be ignored or dismissed, celebrating the mysteries of life, death suffering and joy, embracing the miracles of existence.

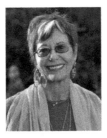

About Jean Watson

Dr. Jean Watson is Distinguished Professor and Dean Emerita, University of Colorado Denver, College of Nursing Anschutz Medical Center campus, where she held the nation's first endowed Chair in Caring Science for 16 years. She is founder of the original Center for Human Caring in Colorado and is a Fellow of the American Academy of Nursing; past President of the National League for Nursing; founding member of International Association in Human Caring and International Caritas Consortium. She is Founder and Director of the non-profit foundation, Watson Caring Science Institute (www.watsoncaringscience.org). In 2013 Dr. Watson was inducted as a Living Legend by the American Academy of Nursing, its highest honor. Her global work has resulted in her being awarded 15 Honorary Doctoral Degrees, 12, international.

As author/co-author of over 30 books on caring, her latest books range from empirical measurements and international research on caring, to new postmodern philosophies of caring and healing, philosophy and science of caring and unitary caring science as sacred science, global advance in caring literacy. Her books have received the American Journal of Nursing's "Book of the Year" award and seek to bridge paradigms as well as point toward transformative models, now, and the future.

For further Lotus Library reading visit our online store: www.watsoncaringscience.org/the-caring-store/